Advance Directives in Mental Health

of related interest

The Nearest Relative Handbook
David Hewitt
ISBN 978 1 84310 522 0

Morals, Rights and Practice in the Human Services
Marie Connolly and Tony Ward
ISBN 978 1 84310 486 5

Ethical Issues in Dementia Care
Making Difficult Decisions
Julian C. Hughes and Clive Baldwin
ISBN 978 1 84310 357 8

Person-Centred Dementia Care
Making Services Better
Dawn Brooker
ISBN 978 1 84310 337 0

Guide to Mental Health for Families and Carers of People with Intellectual Disabilities
Edited by Geraldine Holt, Anastasia Gratsa, Nick Bouras, Theresa Joyce, Mary Jane Spiller and Steve Hardy
ISBN 978 1 84310 277 9

Introducing Mental Health
A Practical Guide
Caroline Kinsella and Connor Kinsella
Foreword by Vikram Patel
ISBN 978 1 84310 260 1

Community Care Practice and the Law
Third edition
Michael Mandelstam
ISBN 978 1 84310 233 5

Good Practice in Adult Mental Health
Edited by Tony Ryan and Jacki Pritchard
ISBN 978 1 84310 217 5

Law, Rights and Disability
Edited by Jeremy Cooper
ISBN 978 1 85302 836 6

Working Ethics
How to Be Fair in a Culturally Complex World
Richard Rowson
ISBN 978 1 85302 750 5

Advance Directives in Mental Health

Theory, Practice and Ethics

Jacqueline M. Atkinson

Jessica Kingsley Publishers
London and Philadelphia

First published in 2007
by Jessica Kingsley Publishers
116 Pentonville Road
London N1 9JB, UK
and
400 Market Street, Suite 400
Philadelphia, PA 19106, USA

www.jkp.com

Library of Congress Cataloging in Publication Data
A CIP catalog record for this book is available from the Library of Congress

British Library Cataloguing in Publication Data
A CIP catalogue record for this book is available from the British Library

ISBN 978 1 84310 483 4

Printed and bound in Great Britain by
Athenaeum Press, Gateshead, Tyne and Wear

Contents

Acknowledgements

Over the last decade or so, many people have listened to me talk about advance directives in mental health. This has included, no doubt, boring my friends (all too good natured to say so), but has also resulted in many interesting and helpful exchanges, discussions and debates. Those to whom I owe a particular debt of gratitude are: Helen Garner and Jacquie Reilly, researchers; Susan Stuart, philosopher; Denise Coia, Roch Cantwell, Donny Lyons, Jim Dyer, psychiatrists; Jenny Graydon (Glasgow Association for Mental Health); Hilary Patrick, lawyer; Mary Weir (National Schizophrenia Fellowship Scotland). I am also indebted to my students over the years in the Master of Community Care class for discussing the topic with so much enthusiasm, and to Heather Savage for administrative and secretarial support. John Dawson at the University of Otago, and finally Marvin Swartz, Jeffery Swanson, Eric Elbogen from Duke University, and Debra Srebnik from the University of Washington were full of interest and support during my visits to them. I am indebted to the Nuffield Foundation for supporting our research and to all the participants in our research projects, and to the service users in all our projects, who have been happy to discuss their ideas with us over the years. I would also like to thank Heta Gylling (previously Heta Häyry) and her publisher, Routledge, for permission to reproduce her 'conditions for the rational person' in Chapter 8.

CHAPTER 1

Introduction: Why Have Advance Directives in Mental Health?

The first thing that is likely to spring to mind when advance directives are mentioned is the phrase 'living will' which situates them, along with the term 'do not resuscitate', at the end of life. The fact that a living will is not restricted to the elderly was brought home to many people when the popular former MP Mo Mowlam died of a brain tumour in 2005 and the existence of her advance directive was made known. In recent years the interest in applying advance directives to mental health has grown, but for many it is still an odd, or alien, concept.

Planning for the future is not, however, an odd concept, and this is the framework in which advance directives are best placed. Whilst the focus is on planning for the time when the person is unable to take competent decisions for themselves, the process is more common than might be apparent. The most obvious example of planning for the future is making a will, with death being the final stage of incapacity. Less dramatic, within a healthcare framework, are birth plans. In this instance it is not that the woman in labour is incompetent to make decisions but a situation in which she needs to set out what she wants to happen at a time when communicating with others might be compromised. For the rich (but not necessarily famous) pre-nuptial agreements can be seen as another form of advance directive.

Most people have, at some time, sought to curb future, less-than-sensible behaviour by making a rash request to a friend or relative. It might not have quite the ring of Olympic Gold Medallist Steve Redgrave's impassioned plea after the 1996 games, having just won his fourth gold medal: 'If anybody sees me near a boat again, please shoot me'. But requests along the lines of 'Don't let me get drunk/eat too much/go home with him or her/buy any more shoes I can't walk in' are understandable. There are times when competence is compromised and some external help is needed.

Advance directives in mental health fall somewhere along this continuum. They may be useful when capacity is lost, and formally judged as such, or they may have a role in managing crises when aspects of capacity are compromised or communication difficult and confused.

However, the issues surrounding advance directives in mental health are complex. How does exercising choice now for the future relate to the person's future choices, which may be different? Steve Redgrave, after all, famously changed his mind about abandoning rowing and went on to win his fifth gold medal. Women in labour change their minds, ask for pain relief and receive it. When is it acceptable to change one's mind? How competent does the person have to be? And if the answer is totally competent, where does that leave the wishes of the person when they have lost capacity or are ill?

These are some of the issues explored in this book. It starts in Part I by looking at influences on the development of interest in advance directives in mental health, first broadly and then more narrowly. Since one of the major concerns of people with major mental health problems is the impact of mental health law on their lives, and the relationship between advance directives and compulsory treatment is complex, influences on mental health law are also considered.

Part II considers some of the philosophical issues which might be seen to underpin advance directives: autonomy, rationality and responsibility, and, most importantly, the concept of the continuity of the person. If priority and power are given to the 'well' person, where does this leave the 'ill' person? It also raises fundamental questions about whether people can choose to stay ill, and whether this can ever be a rational decision.

Part III moves into the practical arena and addresses the issues involved in making an advance directive and their impact on practice, from uptake to outcomes.

These are all wide-ranging issues and, inevitably, it is not possible to do justice to them all within one book. The issue of assessing capacity, for example, is touched on, but really requires a book in its own right. Rather, the author's intention is to bring together a wide variety of approaches to considering advance directives in mental health and introduce these to a broad interdisciplinary audience.

The first half of the twenty-first century is an exciting time for advance directives. They were introduced in Scotland, as advance statements, in the Mental Health (Care and Treatment) (Scotland) Act 2003 in an important and innovative way. An increasing number of states in the USA have developed, or are developing, specialised legislation for psychiatric advance directives. From a slow start there is a growing amount of empirical research to help answer clinical and other questions. The time to take advance directives in mental health seriously has come.

Author's note on language

When an advance directive comes into force the 'person' will, by definition, be a 'patient'. In most cases in current research studies the person is a patient when they make the advance directive. They need not be. Along with this there is the problem some groups have with the term 'patient' in any context, preferring the term 'service user' or 'consumer'. Throughout I have mixed terminology, rather than align to one position, and in many cases use the terminology of those whose work I am discussing.

In the philosophy-based chapters there is a special problem. The words 'mental illness' are used to describe conditions which are not always defined and would not always accord with a clinical diagnosis of mental illness. Some philosophers equate mental illness with madness. For the sake of an abstract discussion, I have chosen to use madness and mad in some of the discussion. I do not intend this to offend anyone (and apologise sincerely if it does) but it is sometimes easier to have an abstract concept of 'madness', which does not really relate to people with mental illness as we know them, than to try to fit clinical frameworks where they were never intended.

PART I

The Context of Advance Directives in Mental Health

CHAPTER 2

Influences on the Development of Advance Directives in Mental Health

The idea of advance directives did not appear out of nowhere. Various factors influenced different groups of people to begin thinking about advance directives and then to come together to develop the idea. This chapter focuses on the social, clinical and political contexts which influenced advance directives and allowed, and even encouraged, their development. Since advance directives are in many ways intimately connected to mental health law, Chapter 3 looks at the background to mental health law. Chapter 4 then considers the development of the directives themselves and the different models.

The various influences were not independent but interacted and fed off one another. Similar issues or ideas might arise in different places at the same time, but under slightly different guises, and move in different directions, only to meet up later on. Even with detailed study it is not always clear who influenced whom, what or when. All have to be set against the changing political and social attitudes of the time. One change saw both Britain and the USA move further to the political right and develop the cult of the individual, a change not noticeably reversed in Britain by subsequent years of New Labour government. Many of the political shibboleths, such as personal choice, social inclusion and greater transparency in government introduced by New Labour, have come up against control issues such as public safety and costs of services.

The influences considered in this chapter are all 'big' topics in their own right and there is no attempt to review them in depth. Rather, the focus is on how, directly or indirectly, they might be seen to provide fertile ground for advance directives. The influences are:

- the development of community care

- the rise of the user movement

- increased concern over stigma and discrimination
- individual responsibility and health
- the framework of control
- the emphasis on personal choice.

Later in this chapter the influence of advance directives in physical health care on the development of advance directives in mental health is reviewed, along with ways in which they might be used to aid understanding and implementation.

The development of community care

The process of deinstitutionalisation and the factors which influenced this have received much analysis and comment, both in Britain and the USA (e.g. Leff 2001; Lewis 1999). Even though there may have been good clinical and human rights reasons to move care to community settings, the cost of running institutions was probably even more important. The way in which community care developed was thus as much a political decision as a clinical one. Thus the model of community care in Britain developed from the political philosophy of Thatcher's Conservative Government and espoused right wing approaches to the individual, responsibility and provision of support services (Atkinson 1994, 1996; Boardman 2005). It was the Griffiths Report (1988), followed by the NHS and Community Care Act 1990 (House of Commons 1990), which introduced not just the focus on services in the community but the purchaser–provider split in the provision of health and social care. This paved the way for voluntary organisations to develop as service providers.

The changing approach to patients – to remodel them as service users, or even consumers – had mixed consequences, or mixed views of consequences. Patient participation was encouraged, whether at national or local level, in developing services, along with involvement in running services through the voluntary organisations, or being employed by these services themselves (often as support workers, befrienders or similar). All this can be seen either as empowering and supportive or limiting and imposed as it still keeps individuals tied to services they may not want (Barnes and Shardlow 1997; Bhui, Aubin and Strathdee 1998; Bowl 1996; Pilgrim 2005; Pilgrim and Waldron 1998; Tait and Lester 2005).

The services run through voluntary organisations and user groups had a different ethos to those run through statutory services. They often interacted more with those who used them, often having users on the management groups. They developed to meet not just local needs, as defined by gaps in the services, but needs as defined by local users.

Some voluntary organisations also took an interest in advocacy and advocacy services. With the support of advocacy workers patients were encouraged and empowered to challenge decisions made by clinicians for them and to take a more active role in decision-making about their treatment, clearly stating their own preferences. Gradually advocacy services moved into the mainstream, including services in the maximum security hospitals (Atkinson and MacPherson 2001). Although funded through the National Health Service (NHS), for the most part advocacy services were run through existing voluntary organisations or new advocacy organisations. Advocacy became such an important aspect of the service users' approach that it was included in the new Mental Health (Care and Treatment) Act in Scotland with widespread support (Atkinson 2006).

With these developments it was natural that some voluntary organisations turned their attention to advance directives (Copeland 2004; Curran and Grimshaw 1999; Manic Depression Fellowship undated; Rethink 2000) as a further way of encouraging service users to engage with, and take control of, their own treatment.

The development of more, and more varied, community-based services and policies, such as the Care Programme Approach (CPA) (Sainsbury Centre for Mental Health 2005), was in part influential in revisions of mental health legislation and the introduction of the controversial Community Treatment Order (CTO) (Atkinson 2006). It was acknowledged that many people, if they took their medication, did not require treatment in hospital, although interventions such as the CPA were described as only being effective 'if service users make a meaningful, not tokenistic, contribution to the process'.

Advance directives would have no impact here unless they were given some legal status that meant they could not be ignored totally by committing someone to detention or compulsory treatment under a mental health act.

The rise of the user movement

Although often referred to in the singular, 'user movement', in many ways it may be more appropriate to refer to the 'users' movements'. The recent history of patients' groups and the transformation into users' movements are most appropriately seen as 'new social movements', occupying a different arena from previous movements which had a focus on labour and the workplace (Habermas 1981). With some influence from the civil rights movement in tackling racism, and with the rise of 'women's liberation', there is a parallel with these movements which are based on oppression through a shared identity. This is in contrast to the 'shared cause movements', such as animal rights or the environmental movement, where disparate individuals have come together through a shared belief. Although many of the common causes of the users' movements may be supported by non-users, there is, for many organisations, a fundamental identity issue at their heart.

There have been three overlapping phases of mental health users' movements in Britain (Crossley 1998). The earliest stems from the organisation of the Mental Patients' Union (Crossley 1999). This was followed by various other groups, and led to Survivors Speak Out being formed in 1986 (Campbell 2005; Crossley and Crossley 2001; Rogers and Pilgrim 1991; Wallcraft, Read and Sweeney 2003).

The diversity of groups has led to what might be seen as 'wings' of the movement. On the radical side there are those who might best be described as protesters or in opposition. This wing has a commitment to patients' or users' rights. It is anti-psychiatry and anti-coercion, but supports user-led services and a self-help agenda. In the USA during the 1970s to mid-1980s there was a range of radical anti-psychiatry groups, including Support Coalition International, the Insane Liberation Front, the Mental Patients' Front and the Network Against Psychiatric Assault (Rissmiller and Rissmiller 2006).

Then there is the less radical and confrontational wing which takes a reformist position. This often actively embraces the participation agenda of community care and recent health policy. Its members may be joined by, or ally themselves with, supportive professionals. Indeed, some health boards have set up their own 'user network' to facilitate involvement and consultation.

The impact of the user voice on service delivery may have its greatest impact through the concept of recovery and what may be seen as the 'recovery movement' (Roberts and Wolfson 2004).The impact of this has been greater in the USA than the UK, where it is, however, gathering momentum, particularly in Scotland. The Scottish Recovery Network is an organisation which promotes this approach, wholly funded by the Scottish Executive (www.scottishrecovery.net).

It would be unfair to suggest a rigid divide between these 'wings', and many groups and organisations embrace people with views from both sides, sometimes in an uneasy alliance. Both 'sides' may support the common cause of opposition to a coercive agenda through compulsory detention in hospital and compulsory treatment and argue for greater choice in treatment and service provision. It is the issue of the legitimacy of psychiatric diagnosis which separates some groups. Both sides may benefit from the changes to service provision that allow voluntary organisations/charities to provide services but the more radical groups may not always find their ideas acceptable or fundable through statutory funders of services.

Users' groups have supported the development of advance directives in mental health, particularly where they allow for the refusal of what would, otherwise, be compulsory treatment. For this reason they are likely to want advance directives to be legally enforceable (Atkinson *et al.* 2003a, 2006; Campbell 1999).

Increased concern over stigma and discrimination

Interest in the impact of stigma and its close companion, discrimination, on health and quality of life has burgeoned in all areas of health in recent years. Although some argue that the particular issues for people with a mental illness stem from the existence of mental health legislation (see Chapter 1) the issues are wider than this (Dunn 1999; Gale and Grove 2005; Read and Baker 1996; Sayce 2000). A number of factors affect the sense of being stigmatised, including the person's experience of stigma or discrimination from others and their history of self-stigmatisation (Hayward and Bright 1997). Advance directives have been suggested as a way of avoiding detention (and compulsory treatment) by opting into treatment. This has been referred to as 'self detention'. The laudable aim of avoiding the stigma of being detained is, however, offset by a number of other problems. This approach does, though, put advance directives in a wider context than the more common 'refusal' approach linked to the advance directive in physical health care.

Individual responsibility and health

The growth of the 'cult' of the individual in the USA and the UK under President Reagan and Prime Minister Thatcher emphasised the importance of an individual's responsibility for, amongst other things, their health and social care. Dependency became a concept derided by the new Right, and the benefits and satisfactions of mutuality, reciprocity and community or societal responsibility seemed to be lost (Atkinson 1994). Thus the Thatcherite vision of community care in Britain was one which took the individual, extended to the family, as the unit of responsibility for care rather than the state.

The focus on the individual was also useful in relating deeply held convictions about autonomy with issues of choice and thus responsibility for choices. One expression of this was seen in the USA in the Patients' Self-Determination Act 1990 which came into practice in 1991 (for a description see Chapter 5). Included within the Act were community mental health centres. Although the position was not always clear, in many states it was made explicit that psychiatric advance directives were allowed (Dunlap 2000–1). As well as emphasising patient autonomy there is an underlying focus in this Act on the patient not only having the right to make such decisions but also on the responsibility to make them.

The years that followed the Labour Government gaining power in Britain have seen responsibility take centre stage in a number of areas, not least in relation to health. Although this is frequently part of the health promotion agenda it goes further. There is an agenda to discuss rationing of treatment and prioritisation of patients for limited procedures where their behaviour or lifestyle, such as smoking, alcohol or diet (Halpern and Barnes 2004; Nuffield Centre on Bioethics 2006) contributed to the illness.

In mental health the issue of responsibility was raised when the political debate got under way in England on the supposed failure of community care and the review of mental health legislation (Atkinson 2006). Patients were seen as being 'responsible', if not for their illness, then for its management, and if they shirked this responsibility they would face coercion. This was summed up by the then Health Minister, Paul Boateng: 'With our safety-plus approach, the law must make it clear that non-compliance with agreed treatment programmes is not an option' (Department of Health 1998). Responsibility was to be enforced.

It could be argued that this provided a perfect backdrop for the development of advance directives which are absolute statements of patients taking responsibility for themselves, not just in the present but also in the future. Interestingly, successive governments in Britain did not pursue this route but concentrated instead on a policy which emphasised patient participation and the development of joint planning through policies such as social work care management and the CPA (Bindman *et al.* 1999; Department of Health 1990, 1995; Simpson, Miller and Powers 2003a, 2003b; Wolfe *et al.* 1997). CPA developed from the case management model in the USA (Ford *et al.* 1993, 1997; Mueser *et al.* 1998; Stein and Test 1980). The involvement of patients through individual planning of their care was separate from the user movement in that it depended on the relationship between the patient and their psychiatrist (or mental health team) and did not require patients to be involved in, or even know about, any wider movement (Anthony and Crawford 2000; Beeforth, Conlan and Graley 1994; Carpenter *et al.* 2004; Lawson, Strickland and Wolfson 1999). Nevertheless, the concept of the 'expert patient' (Chief Medical Officer 2001) replaced, in some quarters, what might have been seen as the oxymoronic 'lay expert' and the acknowledgement that individual patients might well be experts in their own care. This approach was to be developed with people with chronic illness, but seems to be focused more on physical than on mental illness (Kennedy, Rogers and Gately 2005).

The belief that taking medication will, by itself, prevent all risk and negative events (whether to the person or to others) might appear naïve but, nevertheless, it appeared to be the cornerstone of the government's thinking.

Contradictory messages were being issued by the government. On the one hand it advocated participation and responsibility, and on the other the spectre of the CTO and the public safety agenda was removing personal control from patients in respect of their treatment, particularly medication.

The framework of control

A philosophy or policy which emphasises responsibility is also likely to develop a blame culture when things go wrong. It might not be reasonable, or possible, always to 'blame' the person for stopping their medication or exhibiting 'risk behaviour' (or at least, not entirely) and another 'culprit' was needed.

Inevitably this was going to be the psychiatrists. They should have made sure the person took their medication, or taken steps – any steps – if this did not happen. These might have involved enforcing the medication or admitting the person to hospital. They should also, of course, have been accompanied by a thorough risk assessment (again with no understanding of the real limitations of risk assessment).

A number of official pronouncements from the British Government (based on dubious, if any, evidence) claimed that community care had failed. This led to a series of measures, under both Conservative and New Labour Governments, aimed at curtailing the freedom of patients who were deemed 'at risk' and putting more responsibility on psychiatrists to control them (Atkinson 1996, 2006; Boardman 2005). These measures were opposed by stakeholders, not least the psychiatrists themselves, who argued that they were not, and did not want to become, agents of social control.

The government nevertheless pressed this agenda with the consequence that the reform of the Mental Health Act in England has been stalled, compared to Scotland where this agenda of control did not really take off (Atkinson 2006; Fennell 2005; Scott-Moncrieff 2005). Advance directives were discussed in relation to the reform of the legislation but were dropped from the agenda, although they formed part of the new law in Scotland.

The emphasis on personal choice

Personal choice has been alluded to throughout this chapter and is clearly linked intimately to responsibility. Within the NHS patient choice has become something of a watchword with a policy which, in theory, allows patients to choose which hospital they attend for treatment (Department of Health 2004). This choice does not extend to patients attending for psychiatric treatment. Although this would seem to be discriminatory, little has been done to challenge this. The Sainsbury Centre (2006) briefing on 'Choice in Mental Health Care' does not address this, although it covers treatment choices, choices in care planning, service planning and delivery, advance directives and direct payments.

All this is despite the testimony of patients who say that they are routinely refused choice of drug treatment and given very little information. In a survey conducted by three mental health charities (National Schizophrenia Fellowship,

Manic Depression Fellowship and Mind), 2600 (62%) said that they had not been offered a choice of medication. The greatest lack of choice was noted for 'typical antipsychotics' and mood stabilisers (National Schizophrenia Fellowship 2001). Patients with schizophrenia want shared decision-making, particularly for those who have been treated compulsorily, who have negative attitudes towards treatment and who are younger (Hamann *et al*. 2005).

The importance patients attach to choice with regard to their medical treatment is not reflected to the same degree by policy makers (Shumway *et al*. 2003). This discrepancy needs to be addressed in developing a consensus in guidelines for treatment.

Nevertheless, the promotion of personal choice would seem to underpin the concept of advance directives. Indeed, in the USA some templates for advance directives specifically incorporate decisions about which treatment facility the person wants to attend but this is likely to be more problematic in the NHS.

It has been argued that there is more choice for patients in the USA, with a wider variety of services, although this does not always mean that there are more choices of treatment (Goldman 2005).

Advance directives in physical health care

Advance directives in physical health care have developed in range and importance in recent years. At first glance there may seem little difference between advance directives during mental illness and those during physical illness. Both set out to give expression to an individual's wishes at some time in the future when they are unable to make decisions. Apart from special cases (the do-not-resuscitate [DNR] directive) the advance directive usually allows for future acceptance, as well as rejection of treatment. In both cases the person must be competent when making the advance directive. Although various laws cover the making of advance directives for both mental and physical health care these are, in fact, embodiments of a right in common law. Thus any clear, competent, prior expression of a person's wishes should normally be honoured.

Having said this, there are some differences between advance directives in mental and physical health care, although sometimes more apparent than real. This is because it is often assumed that advance directives in physical health are used only for end-of-life situations. In such cases the nature of the decision is seen as different. On the one hand the objective is enabling 'a good death' and on the other in securing 'a good life' (Dresser 1982). Not all advance directives in physical health are for terminal conditions, however, and some, such as birth plans, may not even relate to illness.

Whilst end-of-life decisions will occur only once in each person's life, episodes of mental illness are likely to be repeated. Thus, in the former it is assumed that the person is making a plan for a situation they have yet to experience, and in the latter for a situation with which they may be all too familiar. This need not be the case, though. Some DNR or other living will directives may be prompted by the treatment and experiences of the person during a previous 'near death' episode. Although it is unlikely that many people will rush to make a psychiatric advance directive without having had a prior episode, those who see themselves as particularly at risk (for example through family history) may have more than a passing interest. Some people would argue that advance directives based on experience are more acceptable, or 'make even more sense' (Dunlap 2000–1), than those based on supposition.

The consequences of the advance directive are also based on this difference in the nature of the decision. Refusing treatment in end-of-life situations will usually hasten death. This is assumed to be positive for the person (this is what they wanted; they have a 'good' death) and arguably for medical services and society in general, or for the patient's family, since not only have they respected the person's wishes (and may thus feel some degree of virtue) but also they do not have to pay for (possibly expensive) life-preserving treatment. Beds and services are freed for other patients. This is not the case with all advance directives in physical illness. Jehovah's Witnesses, for example, who refuse blood transfusion, may end up having surgery that is longer and more of a problem for the surgeon than conventional surgery.

Birth plans, as written, formalised documents (rather than informal plans made with family and friends), were introduced in the 1980s in response to the medicalisation of birth and a way of helping women avoid the growing number of interventions deemed 'necessary' (Inch 1988; Kitzinger 1992, 2000; Lothian 2006; Perry, Quinn and Lindemann Nelson 2002). Latterly, however, birth plans are as likely as not to reflect the 'intervention-intensive birth' and request interventions such as epidurals, elective indications and caesarean sections. This is in spite of increasing evidence that many standard practices are unnecessary and, indeed, potentially harmful. The World Health Organisation (World Health Organisation Department of Reproductive Health and Research 1999) recommends that the goal should be the least intervention possible to achieve a healthy mother and child.

Although birth plans are seen as helpful by some women there are no clear differences between women who have one and those who do not in their experience of labour and birth (Brown and Lumley 1998; Lundgren, Berg and Lindmark 2003; Whitford and Hillan 1998).

Lothian (2006) suggested that the purposes of a birth plan are to determine personal expectations, develop relationships with service providers and share decision-making. To this end she suggests a plan which outlines goals such as 'to avoid use of EFM' (electronic foetal monitoring) and then outlines a list of things which the person can do to help achieve this goal. This is something which is mirrored in some approaches to advance planning in mental health and may be seen particularly in joint crisis plans.

There are some striking similarities between many of the developments in and implementation of birth plans and advance directives in mental health. Not least is that many of the tensions in the implementation of birth plans are a reflection of two different 'world views' on labour and birth (Lothian 2006). One is that it is a normal, natural process and that women have an inherent ability to birth their babies. Set against this is that labour and birth are risky and 'the possibility that things could go terribly wrong' requires a management of labour and birth that involves routine monitoring or invasive interventions 'just in case'.

This might be compared with the two world views in mental health. The 'traditional' or medical view of mental illness is an *illness* which requires treatment and interventions, again sometimes with a view as to what might happen or go wrong. The opposing view is that there is no such thing as mental illness, and that distress is best helped and supported by non-medical interventions. Similarly, the outcomes people want to achieve with their birth plan/advance directive may have as much to do with the *process* of reaching the goal as the goal itself.

Refusing treatment for a mental illness is different to physical illness in that it is unlikely to lead to death. It is, however, possible to die from mental illness, and not just through suicide. Severe catatonic depression and extreme hypermania may lead to death if not treated. The person is likely, however, to become more severely ill and to remain ill, and in hospital, for longer than if treated. This has negative consequences for both the individual and for psychiatric services. Thus, although it feels virtuous to respect the person and their autonomy, it is also likely to engender negative feelings at someone who is 'causing more trouble than is necessary' and costing services more money.

A special area of advance directives which straddles physical and mental health is Alzheimer's disease and other dementias. Here, advance directives are similar to physical illness in that the person will not have experienced the situation before and it will probably incorporate end-of-life decisions though these may be some time distant. As with psychiatric advance directives, people are likely to want to cover a much wider range of circumstances than just treatment issues and include, for instance, finances and where the person will live. Another similarity to physical illness is the now incapable person wanting to make decisions which conflict with the advance directive. In some instances these may be seen to make the incapable person's life 'better', although conflicting with previously held views.

Despite this there are some areas where the limited research on advance directives in psychiatric illness can be supplemented by research on advance directives in other areas of health care.

The history of advance directives in physical health care, and living wills in particular, is not wholly positive (Backlar 1997; Dresser 1994; Hoffman, Zimmerman and Tompkins 1996; Levinsky 1996). The number of people making advance directives under the Patient Self-Determination Act is considerably lower than had been hoped for. Some have gone so far as to suggest that since resources have been 'lavished' (p.38) on a policy of making living wills 'routine and even universal' (p.31), and that results have not been forthcoming 'that recompense costs' (p.31), this approach should be 'renounced' (p.39) and the Act repealed (Fagerlin and Schneider 2004).

This may be premature. Molloy *et al.* (2000) found that implementing advance directives systematically in nursing homes reduced the use of health care services and subsequent costs, with no impact on patient satisfaction. It is not clear, however, if appropriate palliative care was provided if the decision was not to admit to hospital (Teno 2000).

CHAPTER 3

Mental Health Legislation

Advance directives in mental health must be seen against the backdrop of mental health legislation. The problem of loss of capacity would still make them necessary even if there were no mental health laws, but the existence of such legislation makes them doubly important, and the need more pressing.

It is easy for views on mental health legislation to become polarised, usually around the autonomy–paternalism axis, but this can, unhelpfully, be oversimplified. The very existence of mental health law sets the scene for relationships between service providers and service users through the provision for compulsory detention and treatment, which regulates these relationships. Where the possibility of compulsion exists the question arises whether voluntary use of services is ever possible.

Whilst it may be quite true that some people with mental health problems fear the way in which the law might be interpreted with regard to their particular position, for most people (e.g. those with mild to moderate depression, anxiety, stress, obsessive compulsive disorders, phobia) it is unlikely that mental health law would ever apply to them. People with more severe mental health problems (or mental illness) may be right to worry, even though most will not be subject to the law. Most people who are detained under mental health law have psychotic disorders, predominantly schizophrenia. The way in which mental health legislation defines mental disorder, including mental illness, is the first safeguard in preventing its indiscriminate use. A series of other criteria must also be met.

The perceived or actual threat of loss of freedom is also cited as a reason for patients not to trust either their psychiatrists or services but the issue of coercion in psychiatric services is outwith the scope of this book. For the moment it is reasonable to assume that the existence of mental health legislation is *perceived* to diminish freedom of choice for a group of patients (size unknown) but *actually* removes choice from a somewhat smaller group.

The presence of compulsory detention and treatment also has an impact on staff, albeit one that is less dramatic. As Unsworth (1987) asserted, mental health law 'Actually constitutes the mental health system...it is indeed a precondition of the intricate mechanisms of control, surveillance, discipline, and reconstruction which assemble into an advanced mental health system' (p.5).

Professionals in mental health services have, unlike other health occupations, a legally defined role which encompasses a duty to exercise a form of social control. This duty – indeed the existence of mental health legislation itself – may be seen as contributing to the stigmatisation of people with mental health problems (Rogers and Pilgrim 1994). Although legislation exists which allows for patients with certain infectious diseases, who are acting in a way which endangers the health of others, to be detained in hospital, it is not possible to treat them against their will if they are competent to refuse.

It is not only mental health legislation which discriminates against people with a mental illness, or indeed, offers protection. The impact of including provisions for people with mental illness in other areas should not be underestimated, either as an expansion or contraction of liberties. A study of all Bills (968) in 2002 in the USA showed provisions for people with mental illness made in all types of health and social service provision from housing to firearms restrictions (Corrigan *et al.* 2005).

Only people who have a mental illness may be treated against their will, although they may be capable of making a decision (e.g. Mental Health Act 1983; Mental Health Act (Scotland) 1984). Although this has recently changed in Scotland and is not necessarily the case in other legal jurisdictions, the fear – or indeed the 'threat' – of being treated against one's wishes is likely to persist for some time. Not unnaturally many people, particularly those likely to be subject to the legislation, have seen it as a method of social control. This aspect cannot be overlooked, but a consideration of the history of mental health law will show that the law has, and has had, a wider remit. Broadly speaking mental health legislation has sought to protect patients from themselves and from others (including exploitation and abuse), to protect the public, and to regulate services (which can be seen as a special case of protecting the patient). These three aspects of the law give rise to a number of tensions, or balancing acts, depending on one's viewpoint:

- protecting the rights and liberties of the individual (the patient) and protecting the public

- protecting the rights of the individual to refuse treatment and the 'right' of the individual to be treated if they are incapable of making that decision

- protecting the individual (the patient) from exploitation or abuse by other individuals (e.g. family and friends) or the wider society (e.g. through discrimination and stigmatisation) and protecting others from the infringement of their rights by people who are mentally ill

- the protection of the patient being detained/compulsorily treated from inappropriate services and the need to deliver services within a resource constrained framework.

The first of these can be summed up as 'protective privilege versus public peril'. This comes from the ruling, on appeal, of the California Supreme Court in the 1975 case of *Tarasoff v. the Regents of the University of California et al.* The decision was that 'protective privilege ends where public peril begins' (quoted by Gurevitz 1977).

The protection of the public (or police power) continues to be high on the agenda, particularly in England (Atkinson 2006) and not only in relation to mentally disordered offenders. This aspect of mental health legislation is not central to a consideration of advance directives in mental health, but it is part of the background. It is ably reviewed by Bean (2001). It will be referred to where relevant but is largely outwith the scope of this book.

The second tension – protecting the rights of the patient – is by no means straightforward. Whilst the law should provide safeguards so that an individual is not inappropriately treated or detained, it also allows the person to be treated against their will, 'in their best interests'. Related to this is consideration capacity, or competence, to make the decision to consent to, or refuse, treatment.

In some states in the USA the preservation of autonomy or the right to refuse treatment has dominated. This has given rise to the expression 'rotting with your rights on' (Gutheil 1980) to describe people who are severely ill, possibly even suicidal, but who refuse treatment, often believing they do not need it. This can be contrasted with *parens patriae* (the state as father) or the public's responsibility to ensure that patients receive appropriate treatment when they are unable to accept treatment for themselves. This 'right to treatment' approach has tended to dominate the legislation in Britain and is the thinking behind the associated incapacity legislation.

Thus the law is trying to walk a tightrope between protecting patients from treatments they do not want, or do not need, and ensuring that those who are unable to consent to treatment, or who pose a risk to themselves, are given the treatment they need. Wherever there is a tightrope it is inevitable that at some point someone will fall. Thus the prudent person might look for a safety net.

The third tension – protecting the person from exploitation or abuse by others – was an early driver, and continues to be an important function, of the law. It has recently seen a strengthening in the new Mental Health (Care and Treatment) (Scotland) Act 2003 (Scottish Parliament 2003).

Whilst no reasonable person would cavil at protecting the vulnerable from exploitation or abuse there is also a need to recognise that the person's family, neighbours or work colleagues should not have their rights infringed unnecessarily by someone who is ill. This might cover general antisocial behaviour, including noise, for which laws or policies might exist. There are two aspects to this. The first is whether the person's behaviour would be subject to external control if it were enacted by someone who was not ill. If the answer is yes, then maybe these measures should be used. The question then arises of how much 'allowance' is made for someone who is ill and may be unable to control their behaviour. Anti-discrimination laws may be of assistance here, including guidance on what is reasonable adjustment.

The second aspect, which is more likely to be of relevance to advance directives, is the expectations placed on families to care for their ill relatives and the 'burden' experienced by them as a result of this. As families have increasingly been expected to take up this role, services have been provided to help them manage the impact on themselves and provide them with knowledge and skills to be more effective in this role. This quasi-professionalisation of family members into carers has brought a number of ethical dilemmas, not least in protecting the patient's confidentiality against the carer's need, sometimes expressed as a right to know, or have, pertinent information (Atkinson and Coia 1989, 1995).

The fourth tension concerns the protection of the patient from inappropriate services. The law provides for the provision of services to voluntary as well as involuntary patients. Although there should be provision for protection of all patients from inappropriate, incompetent, inadequate or abusive services, the main concern for detained and compulsorily treated patients will be the appropriateness and adequacy of services provided in compensation for being deprived of their liberty or freedom of choice. Often referred to as an issue of reciprocity (Eastman 1994), this was recognised as one of the underpinning principles in the Mental Health (Care and Treatment) (Scotland) Act 2003 (Scottish Executive 2001).

Although many of these tensions concern the patient and the professional (often as an agent of the state) there is another, and that is between the professions – doctors and lawyers – for power under the law (Bean 2001; Jones 1991). Thus the balance between each of these results in a law which might be deemed 'good' or 'fair' or 'harsh' or 'coercive' depending on one's stance in relation to the central strands. As with advance directives, what is 'good' or 'bad' is, in many ways, subjective. To place this balance in context, brief consideration will be given to the history of mental health law in Britain.

A brief history of mental health legislation

Before mental illness there was madness. Before there was treatment control and management and before there were hospitals there were workhouses and madhouses. Nevertheless the mad have always been seen as different and, at various times, afforded measures of protection.

The eighteenth century

The English Vagrancy Act 1714 was an 'Act for…the More Effectual Punishing such Rogues, Vagabonds, Sturdy Beggars, and Vagrants, and Sending them Wither They Ought to be Sent'. It authorised 'the furiously mad and dangerous' to be 'safely locked up, in such secure place' for as long as 'such lunacy or madness shall continue' (cited by Porter 1990). This would be authorised by one or two Justices of the Peace. An absence of specialised secure accommodation and any provision for treatment meant that it was unlikely most lunatic vagrants were treated any differently from other vagrants covered by the Acts. They resided in local gaols, workhouses or similar, although the whipping of lunatics was prohibited, unlike other inmates (Porter 1990). Where the lunatic was a pauper the parish paid, otherwise the costs of confinement were met by the lunatic's estate or family. An amendment to the Vagrancy Act in 1744 allowed for dangerous lunatics to be chained. Probably the most important addition to the new Act was the mention of cure. The Act allowed for the 'keeping, maintaining and curing' of the dangerous lunatics in custody.

Whereas current mental health legislation puts a duty on the National Health Service (NHS) and local authorities (LAs) to provide appropriate mental health services, early mental health legislation was more concerned with regulating private provision which was already in existence. There were private madhouses through Britain as well as a few public ones. The oldest is Bethlem Hospital (Bedlam) which had its 750th anniversary in 1997. Some madhouses seem to have had good standards of living and care. Probably the best known is 'The Retreat', founded in York in 1769 by the Quaker merchant, William Tuke. The Retreat popularised the concept of 'moral treatment' and care based on kindness and gentleness. Elsewhere conditions were no better than the workhouses or gaols and abuse was common. Some private madhouses took pauper lunatics from workhouses and it was these people who were most likely to live in the worst conditions (Jones 1991; Parry-Jones 1972).

The rich might well have lived in better conditions in the private madhouses but were subjected to other kinds of abuse. Relatives, with the collusion of the proprietors of the private madhouses, could incarcerate their wealthy but unstable relatives and thus gain control of their money and lands. The only way of freeing such people was through the use of *habeas corpus*. Since, however, there was no requirement for a proprietor to keep records, and patients could be given new names and transferred between madhouses to hide their whereabouts, this was not an effective way of protecting people.

Many physicians and mad-doctors were happy with this arrangement as they were either proprietors or had financial stakes in the private madhouses. The Act for Regulating Private Madhouses 1774 was passed after more than ten years of negotiation. It was the first legislation to police the management of, and trade in, the mad. Its primary aim was to protect the rich, propertied lunatic.

The medical profession gained some power in that all but paupers required a medical practitioner to certify them before legal confinement. This was intended to guard the wealthy sane from being locked away, which had previously been possible. It was assumed that 'henceforth the public should be protected by physicians' integrity, mediating between family and sufferer' (Porter 1990, p.152). Whether this actually protected anyone or merely legalised the *status quo* is debatable.

It may, in some cases, have made release more difficult as the views on insanity by physicians may have carried more weight than those of magistrates. Indeed, this was to become an important goal as 'the doctors now sought to clarify and extend their approved monopoly of the right to define mental health and illness' (Scull 1982, p.151).

The 1774 Act may have done something to protect constitutional liberties but it did little to end the abuse of inmates in private madhouses although it did raise their public profile. What it did do, however, was to collect, for the first time, statistics on how many people were confined, who they were, and where they were. The wherewithal for psychiatric epidemiology was born.

If conditions in the madhouses or workhouses were poor, living in the community did not guarantee better conditions (Jones 1991; Shorter 1997). In 1776 Dr William Perfect visited a maniacal man in Kent confined in a workhouse. 'He was secured to the floor by means of a staple and an iron ring, which was fastened to a pair of fetters about his legs, and he was handcuffed' (quoted by Shorter 1997, p.3). Although madhouses such as Bedlam were well known attractions for the public to view inmates, being in the 'community' brought similar visitors. Perfect's report continues that through the bars of the window 'continual visitors were pointing at, ridiculing and irritating the patient, who was thus made a spectacle of public sport'.

The nineteenth century

These conditions continued into the nineteenth century. In rural Massachusetts in 1840 the pioneering social reformer Dorethea Dix was discovering mad people caged and manacled by both their families at home and also in public almshouses (Dix 1843). Dix found similar conditions when she visited Scotland in 1855 and conditions were no different across the rest of Europe.

Such conditions have to be set against the low standards of living for much of the population at that time. The appalling conditions of damp hovels, without light or sanitation, and piles of refuse in houses and streets, combined with over-crowding, produced an environment where disease was rife. Such conditions are described in detail in Edwin Chadwick's *Report on the Sanitary Conditions of the Labouring Population of Great Britain* (1842). In this he describes people as being 'worse off than wild animals'. Notwithstanding prevailing conditions and the improvement in conditions in the better madhouses, the majority of accounts of madhouses and asylums at this time suggest that conditions were appalling.

The nineteenth century saw a building spree made possible by cheap land prices and labour. A network of both public and private asylums sprang up across the country. The County Asylums Acts of 1808 and 1828 made public money available for the care and maintenance of lunatics. Both Acts introduced statutory requirements for local Justices of the Peace to make visits as well as regulations regarding admissions, discharges and deaths. The 1828 Act had been preceded by two select committees in 1816 and 1827 concerned with abuse.

In Scotland the period between 1781 and 1839 saw the establishment of the seven Royal Asylums. These were privately funded but the Royal Charter required them to accept both rich and poor patients. The Crichton Royal in Dumfries, for example, was founded by Elizabeth Crichton with a donation of £100,000 to build a 120-bed hospital in the 1830s (Shorter 1997).

The 1828 Madhouses Act regulated private madhouses in the London area. It also set up a statutory body, the Metropolitan Commissioners in Lunacy, which was made up of five medical practitioners and 11 Members of Parliament, one of whom, Lord Ashley (later Earl of Shaftsbury 1851), chaired the Commission. They reported to the Secretary of State for the Home Department and had a programme of visits. They were able to recommend the revoking of a licence and could order the immediate release of anyone they believed to be wrongly held. They also developed guidelines for good practice.

In 1832 an amendment to the Act specified that two of the Commissioners must be barristers. Lord Ashley continued to maintain, in 1842, that there was no need for any of the Commissioners to be medically qualified. He argued:

> Although so far as health was concerned the opinion of a medical man was of the greatest importance, yet it having been once established that the insanity of the patient did not arise from the state of his bodily health, a man of common sense could give as good an opinion as any medical man he knew (respecting his treatment and the question of his sanity) (quoted by Scull 1982, p.152).

This mix of law and medicine, assisted by lay people, has remained ever since, apart from the period following the 1959 Mental Health Act until its amendment in 1983. The Metropolitan Commissioners in Lunacy were the forerunners of the present day Mental Health Act Commission in England and Wales and the Mental Welfare Commission for Scotland.

Lord Ashley's reforming zeal led, in 1842, to a national inquiry with the concerns about lack of accommodation for the insane and pauper lunatics being sent so late that any hope of improving their condition was unlikely. The report was published in 1844 and led to two Acts in 1845, the Lunatics Care and Treatment Act and the Lunatics Asylum Act, which together formed the first comprehensive mental health law.

Every county and borough in England and Wales now had a statutory obligation to provide, at public expense, accommodation for its pauper lunatics (Scull 1982). The first 20 years after the Act saw a decline in the number of patients in private madhouses as the number of county asylum beds grew from 8000 to 25,000, bringing in patients previously housed in gaols and workhouses (Jones 1991). Non-medically run asylums were being driven out by the power of the medical profession.

The Lunacy Commission was established with jurisdiction over the whole country (England and Wales) and their remit extended to both private madhouses and the county and London asylums. It included a mix of lay members, including Lord Ashley in the chair, medical and legal commissioners.

Although these Acts can be seen as trying to improve the lot of lunatics by regulating the conditions in which they were kept and regulating who could be confined, there were still discriminatory practices between the rich and the poor. These legal and administrative differences suggest that the certification of madness was as much, if not more, a social and financial classification as it was a medical one. There was also a gender imbalance, and by the 1850s there were more women than men in asylums (Showalter 1987).

At the same time as the number of women inmates was rising the role of women as proprietors was diminishing and was phased out as medicine took hold. Previously up to a quarter of private madhouses were licensed to women. Since women were unable to study medicine at this time they were unable to take up licences for public asylums and were discouraged from applying (Showalter 1987).

During the 1860s and 1870s there was a concern among the general public about both the lunacy law and asylums. The spread of disquiet was aided by the popularity of the first cheap newspapers and the desire, then as now, for promoting readership by publishing sensational stories. Despite some of the evidence being outdated, two Select Committees of the House of Commons, in 1859 and 1877, demanded that Lord Shaftsbury defend the Lunacy Commission. Shaftsbury, along with many asylum doctors, argued, as many still do, that what was most important was not a change in the law, but greater public support, as well as better staff and staff training.

Amid this unease the Alleged Lunatics' Friend Society was founded. The group counted among its members former asylum patients as well as members of the Establishment (Jones 1991). The Society was not concerned with the welfare of lunatics who were incarcerated but with preventing people being committed to asylums. It campaigned for the two mandatory medical certificates for detention to be supplemented by a magistrate's order before a patient could be detained.

It was not until the Lunacy Act of 1890 (six years after the death of Lord Shaftsbury) that the safeguards demanded by the legal profession were introduced, against medical opinion. Porter (1990) described the effect of this Act as 'to straightjacket patients, doctors and magistrates alike' (p.11).

The 1890 Lunacy Act ran to 342 sections and sought to leave nothing to chance, nor to the discretion of the medical profession. Different kinds of order allowed for treatments of different duration. Importantly it sought to prevent inappropriate admission by prohibiting certain forms of relationship between the two certifying doctors, between doctors and institution owners/managers and between doctors and patients (Jones 1991).

The Act gave precedence to lawyers rather than doctors in the management of the mad. Treatment was controlled by law, a matter of last resort rather than the offer of help and prevention of deterioration for which doctors had been fighting. The doctors believed that such measures would delay treatment and deter patients from seeking treatment. Their preferred option had been to move to greater informality so that treatment could be started earlier and on an informal basis. Jones (1991) described the Act as setting 'the treatment of mental illness back for many decades' (p.96).

The twentieth century

For the next 69 years this was the legislation that governed the treatment of the mentally ill in England and Wales. Several pieces of legislation, however, modified the Act before it was swept away in 1959. The first was to establish the difference in law between the feeble-minded or mentally deficient and those who were mad or mentally ill. The former were removed from the Act. The second followed another period of campaigning. The Alleged Lunatics' Friend Society had been succeeded by the National Society for Lunacy which campaigned for reform and was still seeking to change the law.

The Report of the Royal Commission on Lunacy and Mental Disorder (1926) framed the recommendations for the Mental Treatment Act 1930. This took the revolutionary view that protecting patients' rights was best accomplished not by further changes to the law to safeguard against unlawful detention but by making provision for both voluntary admission and discharge.

This Act was historic in protecting the rights of the mentally disordered. Not only was voluntary treatment introduced but so was outpatient treatment. The way was paved for voluntary (in the 1959 Act to become informal) patients to outnumber involuntary (or formal) patients. The 1890 Act, however, remained in place with the assumption that it would fade from use.

The third piece of legislation that modified the 1890 Act was the reorganisation of the delivery of health services following the National Health Act of 1946. This saw mental health services integrated into mainstream medicine, although not without a fight. In the plans of 1943 mental health services were explicitly excluded by the Ministry of Health, only for there to be a U-turn the following year.

It is clear that by the 1950s the 1890 Act had run its course. Still popular with those who wanted no discretion and every contingency prescribed for, it had become a legal mess and a relic of a former way of viewing mental illness. Terminology reflected the move to viewing mental illness as a medical not legal condition: patients had replaced inmates, attendants had become nurses and asylums were now hospitals. Both the agencies and the services had changed, making large sections of the Act irrelevant and/or superseded by later legislation. Medicine had triumphed over law. Mental illness was now a medical, not a legal, problem (Jones 1991).

The Percy Commission was set up and reported in 1957. The Board of Control (which had replaced the Lunacy Commission), overwhelmed by numbers and the weight of documentation, recommended its own abolition and replacement with visitation by Regional Hospital Boards. The mental health system was to be freed from its many constraints so that it could respond freely to the changing needs of patients.

The Mental Health Act 1959 (there was a similar Act in Scotland in 1960) repealed 70 other Acts and amended a further 60. It was noteworthy for introducing the concept of community care. The main concern of the legislation was to make this new service workable rather than protecting the liberty of the mentally ill. This was to be left to the new Mental Health Review Tribunal, a three-person panel comprising one lay, one medical and one legal member. This tribunal would hear appeals by patients against detention. In Scotland, however, both detention and appeal were left in the hands of the Sheriffs.

The ink on the Act was barely dry and the dust had not yet settled when the revisionist legal view reasserted itself. The 1960s saw the emergence of the so-called anti-psychiatry movement. Although many rejected the label, and there were some wide differences of medical and political opinion among them, they set out the case against psychiatry as practised by the medical profession. The leaders were primarily the psychiatrist R.D. Laing in Britain, Irving Goffman and

Thomas Szasz in the USA, and Michel Foucault in Europe. These people largely rejected the concept of mental illness as an 'illness' like physical illness. Behaviour which had been diagnosed as an illness was being redrawn as everything from straightforwardly antisocial to understandable in the face of an insane society. It was seen as resulting from everything from pressure by families to pressure by capitalist governments. The 'medical model', so long fought for and so recently won, was rejected as a form of social engineering and social control.

Contributing to the debate were escalating numbers of allegations of ill treatment in hospitals and a series of national scandals in hospitals in the early 1970s. By now over 90 per cent of patients had informal status yet it was concern over detention as well as abuse by staff which fuelled the media reports, both in newspapers and on television. In the USA, however, the majority of the patients were still compulsorily detained. This preoccupation and their methods were transported to Britain, despite the differences in the systems and in the patient populations.

The American Civil Liberties Union was very active and sought to introduce the principles of 'due process' into the mental health services. This was fostered in Britain, particularly by Larry Gostin. MIND, the campaigning mental health charity, appointed the American Gostin, a recent law graduate with civil rights experience, as their Legal and Welfare Rights Officer. They began a campaign to change the law, particularly to limit the powers of psychiatrists. Gostin set out a detailed critique of the problems and outlined his proposals in his book *The Human Condition* (1975).

Meanwhile treatments themselves were coming under attack. The very drugs which contributed to the possibility of care in the community were also seen as means whereby psychiatrists could control behaviour which was not necessarily ill, just inconvenient. Electro-convulsive therapy (ECT) and psychosurgery were even more feared forms of social control.

All these pressures, coming at the same time, confirmed the need for a new independent statutory body to protect patients' rights. The Board of Control had been premature in declaring itself redundant. From a debate conducted by and large through the media the Mental Health Act (1983) was born. (There was a similar Act in Scotland in 1984.) This Act was closer to the spirit of the 1890 Act in that doctors and mental health officers again operated within a detailed set of prescriptive Sections for detaining patients.

The Board of Control reappeared, now named the Mental Health Act Commission. As well as the usual medical, legal and lay members, there were members from other professions. The Chair of the Commission was a lawyer. The Mental Welfare Commission for Scotland was similar. The latter saw its responsibilities extended in the Mental Health (Care and Treatment) (Scotland) Act 2003. Both Commissions visit hospitals and comment on conditions but their primary purpose is to ensure that patients are aware of their rights. Both issue public reports, highlighting areas of concern as well as reporting statistics on detained patients.

Despite the revisions of the 1983 Act in England and Wales and the 1984 Act in Scotland, both were still in essence the 1959/1960 Acts with some modifications. Provision of services had changed, and would change further during the 1980s and 1990s with a greater emphasis on community care. The law, however, was firmly focused on treatment in hospital. A number of incidents in the community prompted political response and intervention and led to the Mental Health (Patients in the Community) Act 1995, which introduced new community provision of supervised discharge orders in England and Wales and community care orders in Scotland (Atkinson 2006). The 1995 Act was only intended to modify what were seen as outdated aspects of the 1983/1984 Acts and was apparently a temporary measure. It was clear that a new, revisionary approach to mental health legislation was needed.

The twenty-first century

In the past the law in Scotland had followed the law in England and Wales, both in time and in its broad approach and conditions. This was about to be overturned. In 1997 the population of Scotland voted in favour of devolution, and the Scottish Parliament was reconvened in 1999. The way was set for England and Wales to develop different approaches to social welfare, including mental health law (Atkinson 2006).

Despite the committee of review being set up in England in 1998 and in Scotland in 1999, Scotland achieved a new law before England. The Mental Health (Care and Treatment) (Scotland) Act was passed by the Scottish Parliament in March 2003 and came into effect in October 2005 (Scottish Parliament 2003).

The Bill in England continues to be challenged, both within Parliament and from without. The House of Lords and House of Commons Joint Scrutiny Committee on the Draft Mental Health Bill (2005) was critical. The Chair of the Scrutiny Committee, Lord Carlile of Berriew QC, in a rebuttal to the government's response (Department of Health 2005), asked Parliament to 'look with analytical determination at the report of their own Scrutiny Committee', pointing out that: 'There is unlikely to be another major legislative slot for compulsory mental health powers in the next 20 years. This opportunity must not be wasted' (Carlile 2005, p.109).

In January 2007 there was still widespread opposition to the third version of the Bill before Parliament (Dyer 2007). The concerns remained as they have been all along: the implications for service users' rights and the perceived obligations on professionals to act as agents of social control. As of June 2007, ammendments were being debated in the House of Lords.

One reason for this difference was the agenda of the Parliaments in influencing the reform process and the drafting of Bills. In Scotland the report of the Millan Committee (Scottish Executive 2001) was largely accepted by Parliament with an emphasis on safeguarding patients' rights and promoting participation. These were set out in a list of ten underlying principles. Public safety was not ignored but it did not take centre stage as in England.

In England, Parliament focused on the public safety agenda, fuelled by the media, to the apparent exclusion of other considerations. The Richardson Committee Report (Department of Health 1999) (similar in many ways to the Millan Committee Report) was largely rejected and a very different Bill drafted. In Scotland the new Act makes a number of major changes:

- It introduces a form of capacity criteria for detention and compulsory treatment.

- It introduces the Mental Health Tribunal for Scotland which replaces the Sheriff court for both detention/compulsory treatment decisions and appeals.

- It introduces community-based compulsory treatment orders (CB-CTOs).

- It introduces the right of access to advocacy services.

- It introduces new criminal offences for people who abuse/exploit people with a mental disorder.

- It takes away the need for relatives to be involved in the detention process but gives them added rights to be consulted and informed and introduces advance statements (their term for advance directives).

CHAPTER 4

Models of Advance Directives: the History of an Idea

At its simplest, the concept of an advance directive is that, when well (capable/competent), a person indicates what they want to happen to them when they are ill and, crucially, not capable of making that decision for themselves. If the person is ill, and has the capacity to make a decision, then there is no need for an advance directive. Thus advance directives serve to 'restore the voice and control of an individual in crisis at a time when they are most needed and yet most often disregarded' (Priaulx 2003).

As might be expected from the various influences on the development of advance directives in mental health there is a variety of terminologies. Although often used interchangeably, some terms imply different approaches, or influences, and it is as well to be clear about the terms and their underlying philosophies.

This chapter will explore the different terms as they relate to different models of advance directives and the different dimensions within models of advance directives. An important qualification is necessary before the models are described. Although psychiatric advance directives, neatly abbreviated to PADs, is a useful generic term, it is not without problems. Currently, it really has currency only in the USA. Although different states have different requirements Swanson *et al.* (2006a) asserted: 'PADs provide two legal devices – mental health advance instructions and proxy decision makers – that can be used separately or together' (p.385).

Since in other legal jurisdictions (e.g. Britain) the option of a proxy is not available, the term 'advance directive for mental health' (or mental health advance directive) is preferred as the generic term. There are various names for the appointed decision-making agent and the generic term 'proxy' will be used throughout this chapter as a general description. The discussion of many of the issues applies to both, although to cover the widest range, advance directive will usually refer to a set of advance instructions.

Terminology and definitions

There is a wealth of terms in the lexicography of advance directives. They include: advance directives, advance refusals, advance statements, advance agreements, psychiatric advance directives (PADs), psychiatric wills, Mill's will, the Ulysses contract, the voluntary commitment contract and the Nexum contract.

The year 1982 saw a sudden rush of publications in the USA on advance directives in mental health which, although small in number, indicated that here was an idea whose time had come and was about to be thrust, if not centre stage, at least *onto* the stage in a supporting role. One of these was the paper, *The psychiatric will: a new mechanism for protecting persons against 'psychosis' and psychiatry*, by Thomas Szasz, published in July 1982. Szasz was already well known for his railing against psychiatry and his dismissal of the concept of mental disease as put forward in a number of popular books (e.g. Szasz 1961, 1963, 1979).

The psychiatric will

Mental illness, Szasz argued, was a label given to behaviours which are unwanted or undesirable or prohibited or feared (Szasz 1961) and for which there are no treatments (Szasz 1979). He did not, however, object to psychological or psychiatric interventions between 'consenting adults' (Szasz 1979). To this end he proposed the idea of the 'psychiatric will', resting on the same principles as those governing the 'ancient practice' of the last will and testament and the more recent invention of the living will. He specifically cited 'the rejection by Jehovah's Witnesses of blood transfusion as a medical treatment' as part of his model (Szasz 1982).

To understand fully what Szasz was proposing we need to comprehend more than just the concept, and see it in the context of his wider thinking and the powerful polemical language he used. Thus:

> The imagery of 'sudden madness' or 'acute psychosis'...represents the dreaded situation that some persons may want to anticipate and plan for. Since involuntary psychiatric confinement is a tradition-honoured custom in modern societies, the situation such persons need to anticipate must be their own sudden madness managed by others by means of commitment and coerced treatment. To forestall such an event, we need a mechanism enabling anyone reaching the age of maturity, who so desires, to execute a 'psychiatric will' prohibiting his or her confinement in a mental hospital or his or her involuntary treatment for mental illness (Szasz 1982, p.768).

This vision of an advance directive goes beyond most other descriptions, which stop short of allowing someone to opt out of involuntary confinement. He argued that the routine use of pre-trial psychiatric examination to determine competence to stand trial would have to be abandoned as 'this tactic could only be used with the permission of the accused'. Along with the presumption of innocence would be the presumption of sanity. As he argued almost 20 years earlier, those who were found guilty of a crime would be punished, and not diverted into the psychiatric system of care and 'treatment' (Szasz 1963).

He sums up the position in the abstract of the 1982 paper thus:

> Individuals who dread the power of psychosis and desire protection from it by embracing, in case of 'need', the use of involuntary psychiatric interventions could execute a psychiatric will in helping with their beliefs. Individuals who dread the power of psychiatry and desire protection from it by rejecting, regardless of 'need', the use of involuntary psychiatric interventions could execute a psychiatric will in keeping with their beliefs. Thus no one who believes in psychiatric protectionism would be deprived of its alleged benefits, while no one who disbelieves in it would be subjected to its policies and practices against his or her will (Szasz 1982, p.762).

Thus, Szasz argued, the psychiatric will protected the person or 'potential future patient' from both coercion and psychiatric neglect, but also protected the psychiatrist from the 'Catch 22' type situation of being sued either for detaining someone or treating them compulsorily or for not detaining them or compulsorily treating them. Few others have been quite so radical in their approach to advance directives, although Szasz's views may resonate with some service users.

Ulysses contract

The year 1982 also saw the expansion of the idea of 'voluntary commitment' (Howell, Diamond and Winkler 1982). A 'precommitment contract' suggested by Howell et al. (1982) could only be made by a person who had a recurrent and treatable psychotic condition. In this were included bipolar disorder, recurrent mania, psychotic depression, but only certain forms of schizophrenia. The previous year Culver and Gert (1981) had used the terms 'Odysseus pact' and 'Odysseus transfer' and in 1982 both Winston et al. and Dresser described Ulysses contracts. It is not clear why the Roman version of the name has been favoured over the Greek, but this has become the name of choice. Elsewhere the term Ulysses directive has been used (Ritchie, Sklar and Steiner 1998) although this is also taken to indicate a Ulysses contract authorised by statute (Cuca 1993).

Ulysses contracts usually have two controversial aspects. First, they are opt-in directives, or advance agreements to be treated, and second, they are irrevocable. Some people see both aspects as relating to Ulysses contracts and others only one. Stavis (1993) saw the 'Ulysses provision' as one simply of opting in to treatment. This can cause some confusion when the irrevocability aspect is taken as primary and also applied to advance refusals.

The attraction of the Ulysses contract for many is as an opt-in directive which allows a person to manage their illness, even though, when ill, they refused treatment. Thus a person who knew they responded to treatment (in these early discussions this would always involve hospital admission for treatment), and also recognised that when ill they would refuse treatment, could 'self-bind' themselves to treatment by a Ulysses contract. They are thus assenting to treatment for some future relapse, this anticipatory consent to be treated as contemporaneous consent. The reasons why people might want to self-bind or self-commit might include feeling that they have more control over the process; that they might be admitted to hospital earlier and gain treatment earlier than if they had to wait to deteriorate to a point where involuntary commitment would be inevitable; that they might gain treatment and admission when ill where the law might not sanction involuntary commitment or to avoid the stigma of involuntary commitment.

For some the very name indicates that the Ulysses contract is irrevocable (Dunlap 2000–1), although this would usually mean irrevocable by the incompetent person. It would be extreme and unusual not to allow such a contract to be changed by a competent person. In some jurisdictions, however, some statutes for advance directives, including durable power of attorney, allow for the directive to be revoked, regardless of the person's competence (Dunlap 2000–1). These two aspects of the Ulysses contract have caused considerable controversy, particularly the relationship between autonomy, personal identity and temporary incompetence, and the relationship between the 'well person' and the 'ill person'. These themes will be dealt with in more detail throughout this book.

Whilst the Ulysses contract was debated in the USA it was a reality in parts of Scandinavia (Elsler 1979). The Norwegian 'law of psychic health protection' allowed a person to commit themselves to an 'irreversible admission' to a psychiatric hospital, which in practice meant the person was not allowed to leave for three weeks, even if they wanted to and changed their minds about their previous instructions. Again this provision only applied to people with a pre-existing, recurring mental illness. A similar provision was available in Denmark.

The Norwegian position notwithstanding, the main interest in opt-in advance directives, and in particular the use of the term Ulysses contract, has remained firmly in the USA (e.g. Backlar 1995; Rosenson and Kasten 1991). The term has not been used in Britain and the opt-in directive has, until recently, excited little interest.

Concern has been expressed as to the relationship Ulysses directives create between the patient, the psychiatrist and the state (Dresser 1982). In most cases psychiatrists are cast as the crew, their role to do the patient's (Ulysses') bidding. A different relationship has been envisioned, however, whereby psychiatrists could be likened to Circe, rather than the ship's crew (Atkinson 2004). In the Greek legend Ulysses asks the advice of Circe, a sorceress, as to the best way to traverse the Sirens safely. It is her wise counsel that guides his actions. In similar view it may be that the advice given by the psychiatrist guides the patient in making a Ulysses contract. This raises another of the major themes in developing models of advance directives: whether they are independently or co-operatively made.

A slightly different take is that of Rosenson and Kasten (1991) who focus on a different part of the story. They suggest that the 'voices that torment the schizo-phrenic patient are analogous to those of the Sirens designed to lure Ulysses to his destruction' (p.2). This is a more than trivial distinction as, like Ulysses, some patients may wish to experience their voices (or other aspects of the psychotic episode) but in a way which keeps them safe from harm (Atkinson 2004). Ulysses asked to be kept safe, by being tied to the mast (an opt-in directive) but not to make use of measures (wax in his ears) which would have prevented the 'problem' (an opt-out directive).

Mill's will

The term 'Mill's will' was advocated by Rogers and Centifanti (1991), who are both 'consumers of mental health services' and advocates. They take issue with the Ulysses contract, as proposed by Rosenson and Kasten (1991), which includes a health care proxy for its 'unstated assumption' that such directives will be in favour of treatment, and point to criticisms of Ulysses contracts on the basis of 'self-paternalism'. They also take issue with Szasz's psychiatric will (despite noting that it allows patients both to refuse and accept treatment).

Looking to John Stuart Mill (1806–1873) for historical authority they note his position on self-determination. Writing in *On Liberty*, published in 1859, Mill stated that:

> The only purpose for which power can be rightfully exercised over any member of a civilised community against his will is to prevent harm to others. His own good, either physical or mental, is not a sufficient warrant. He cannot rightfully be compelled to do so or forbear because it will make him happier, because, in the opinion of others, to do so would be wise, or even right (Mill 1859/1969, p.135).

Of course, Mill continues in the next paragraph to say that:

> It is perhaps hardly necessary to say that this doctrine is meant to apply only to human beings in the maturity of their faculties... Those who are still in a state to require being taken care of by others must be protected against their own actions as well as against external injury (p.135).

It is not clear that Rogers and Centifanti only intend a Mill's will to be used in cases of expected harm to others. They do, however, draw on another of Mill's concerns, that of an individual giving up their rights in advance and selling themselves into slavery.

> The reason for not interfering, unless for the sake of others, with a person's voluntary acts, is consideration for his liberty. His voluntary choice is evidence that what he so chooses is desirable, or at least endurable, to him, and his good is on the whole best provided for by allowing him to take his own means of pursuing it. But by selling himself for a slave, he abdicates his liberty; he forgoes any future use of it beyond that single act…he is no longer free…the principle of freedom cannot require that he should be free not to be free (p.236).

The advance consent to treatment aspect of the Ulysses contract has been likened to consenting to give up future freedom. To this end the Mill's will proposal included both the right to refuse treatment and to accept treatment. Rogers and Centifanti suggest that it should form a 'written record of our choices' which should include 'a recital of our treatment choices, both pro and con, our related treatment history, a statement of our understanding of our rights to choose and refuse, and some expression of our concerns about not having our wishes overridden or ignored' (Rogers and Centifanti 1991, p.13).

Rogers and Centifanti also suggest the usefulness of naming choices of 'legal council or advocate' and 'our choice – or opposition to – particular treatment venues'.

The involvement of clinicians and lawyers in drafting the Mill's will is advocated, along with family and friends as witnesses. A function of the latter is to bear witness as to competency, wishes and underlying reasons should the Mill's will be challenged.

In arguing 'why the Mill's will has a better chance to work than either the Ulysses or psychiatric will' Rogers and Centifanti point to having it drafted and defended by an attorney or advocate but persist in seeing the other two options as straightforward acceptance or refusal of treatment, which is not the case.

Advance directives and psychiatric advance directives

Although the advance directive is probably the most commonly used term it also has the most meanings. It can be used as a 'catch-all' or generic term to incorporate the other terms or as a specific term or model in its own right. Winick (1996), for example, uses 'advance directive instruments' as 'a general term that includes both health care instruction directives, and health care proxies and powers of attorney' (p.60). Where an advance directive includes both aspects the directive (usually written) from the person is usually referred to as an 'advance instruction'.

In Britain the advance directive has been equated, in general medicine at least, with advance refusal (Department for Constitutional Affairs 2003) and is often taken as synonymous with either a living will or a 'do not resuscitate' (DNR) order. The term psychiatric advance directive (PAD) has been introduced in much of the USA, presumably to indicate what potential situation it covers. Whether there is any real difference between, or need to separate, an advance directive in psychiatry and one in any other branch of medicine is open to debate. It does have a legal meaning in some places and not others.

Definitions of mental health advance directives tend to be fairly straightforward, where they are given, but it should be noted that many authors use the term with implicit rather than explicit understanding of what is meant. Examples of descriptions, rather than definitions, include:

> A psychiatric advance directive (PAD), like a living will, allows a person, anticipated at some time in the future to lack the capacity to make treatment decisions, to make choices while they do have the capacity, when capacity is later lost, the PAD has the same validity as a decision made contemporaneously (Sullivan and Szmuckler 2001, p.1).

> A mental health advance directive (MHAD) is a written document that describes your directions and preferences for treatment and care during times when you are having difficulty communicating and making decisions. It can inform others about what treatment you want or don't want, and it can identify a person called an 'agent' who you trust to make decisions and act on your behalf (Washington State Department of Social and Health Services 2004).

Elsewhere the potential for confusion is added to by advance directives being used for other types of forward planning. Thus: 'An advance directive is like having the living will of mental health. You may have heard it referred to as a Crisis Plan' (Copeland 2004). Crisis plans may be more like advance agreements.

Advance statements

A linguistic nicety might suggest that advance statements are a slightly weaker version of advance directives in that they state the person's wishes rather than direct the other to action. It is not a commonly used term but it is the preferred term in Scotland, being introduced in the Mental Health (Care and Treatment) (Scotland) Act 2003. It is not clear why this term is preferred to advance directive, which has greater international currency, but it separates it as a concept from advance directives in physical illness.

Elsewhere advance statement has been used only as the generic term, where advance directive only refers to an advance refusal (Department for Constitutional Affairs 2003).

Advance agreements

Advance agreements may be seen by some as the weakest form of advance directive as they require an agreement between the person making the directive and those who will implement it. The freedom for the person to express fully their autonomous wishes is thus clearly compromised. Many choices may not be available, including refusing all or certain treatments, if these have to be agreed with the treating (or other) psychiatrist. Other concerns may be with both service or treatment availability and the impact of the agreement on services. It may also be that the person is discouraged from taking risks, for example by stopping treatment, which may lead to consequences with which the doctor does not want to deal.

The discussions leading to the advance agreement may help improve communication or, indeed, the relationship between the patient and the doctor but this is at the expense of the patient's autonomy. It could be argued, however, that in the long term an improved relationship with the treating doctor may lead to a better understanding by the psychiatrist of the patient's position and thus a greater willingness to consider the patient's views.

It is self-evident that the person making an advance agreement will have had to have been ill, and have a recurring illness, as there needs to be an appropriate clinician with whom to make the agreement.

In some circumstances advance agreements may resemble joint crisis plans. Indeed, a study of the latter (Henderson *et al.* 2004) was proclaimed as '*advance agreements*' on the cover of the *British Medical Journal* in which the article appeared. The authors, however, were clear that what they were describing was not an advance directive.

Another hybrid, which may fit under an advance agreement, was the 'Preference for Care' booklet devised by Papageorgiou *et al.* (2002). Although described by the authors as an advance directive, it may be seen as an advance agreement as it had to be agreed with someone, even though that person was described as 'independent'. The booklet required the patient to complete a series of seven statements. This may have influenced patients to think and complete their choices in a particular way.

Nexum contract

Stavis (1999) proposes the term 'Nexum contract' for an advance agreement making use of the Latin word used in Roman law for the first recognised contract. In this case the advance agreement follows a clearly 'contractual model' in that it is 'inherently bilateral'. Not only is the patient committed to the treatment of their choice, but it also commits the 'treatment system to the patient'. Provision is made for a 'well-regarded mandatory arbitration system.'

Dimensions of advance directives

There are a number of dimensions on which to base models of advance directives. These include:

- weak–strong (or legally binding or not)
- opt-in and opt-out directives
- the content of directives (medical treatment only or wider)
- independent or co-operative directives
- the intended outcome.

Weak–strong dimensions

This dimension essentially concerns how binding the advance directive is on treating clinicians (and possibly others) – in other words their status in law.

The drive for legally binding advance directives comes, not surprisingly, from patients and service users and their representative groups. Many have suggested that there is no point in having advance directives unless they are legally enforceable, as they believe that without this psychiatrists will routinely overturn them. Although there is little research in this area this somewhat jaundiced view might be true. The case of *Hargreaves v. Vermont* (Appelbaum 2004), which upheld a person's right not to be treated, indicated that some psychiatrists at least are uncomfortable with not being able to treat a patient who has refused treatment.

Not all patients who want legally binding advance directives do so because they want to refuse treatment. Some do so to ensure that they receive treatment when they need it.

What is it that makes the psychiatrist so uncomfortable? There are several possible reasons. The first might be considered as 'the drive to do good'. Doctors are trained to do good: the Hippocratic oath states 'first do not harm'. Even though medical schools include more and more medical ethics in the curriculum on issues such as autonomy, consent and choice, the traditional emphasis on vanquishing illness and disease remains. It should not be surprising, therefore, that many doctors find it difficult to distance themselves from this training and accept that not everyone wants treatment. This is neither to support, excuse nor rationalise their position but to put it in a context which has to be addressed if advance directives are to be taken seriously.

Allied to this is the second reason – that of clinical autonomy. Consultants expect to be able to exercise their own clinical judgement without interference as the best treatment for a patient (although increasingly within clinical standards frameworks and best practice guidelines). An advance statement challenges this clinical autonomy and doctors may feel frustrated or impotent when prevented from using that clinical judgement to provide what they believe to be the best treatment and clinical care. As practices involving partnership working with patients and increasing self-management by patients take hold, doctors may find it easier to accept this aspect of advance directives when framed as advance agreements.

It should also be noted that nowhere does an advance directive, even if legally binding, expect a doctor to provide any treatment, including medication, against their clinical judgement. It is highly unlikely that a point will be reached where patients will be allowed to demand and receive whatever treatment they choose.

A third reason may have to do with the imposed responsibility on the doctor in caring for someone who is refusing treatment, and was highlighted in the study by Atkinson, Garner and Gilmore (2003b). Although the doctor may not be held responsible for the medical consequences of refusal to treat (and the law usually makes this clear) the treating team still has to keep not only the patient safe, but also other patients and staff. This might not be easy and might involve, in more extreme cases, containment methods staff would prefer not to use, such as restraints and seclusion (Atkinson 2006). In both this and other circumstances where the person is near death, doctors may be concerned not just about being held responsible for a negative outcome but also about litigation from the patient's family.

The fourth reason is likely to relate to the impact on services. People who refuse treatment but who are either detained in hospital or voluntarily agree to stay in hospital untreated may be seen as taking up a bed which may be 'better' used by someone who wants to be treated. Especially where someone is detained and they have been in hospital for a longer than usual time this may be perceived as inappropriate (or even selfish) bed blocking, leading to a secondary service for voluntary patients.

Other reasons for not having a legally binding advance directive include concerns about patients requesting services which are not available, whether on the National Health Service (NHS) in general or in the locality. Some of this depends on what is allowed in an advance directive and on local service delivery. Thus in some states in the USA it might be possible to specify which hospital/treatment facility the person wants to be admitted to, and have this honoured by their insurance, whereas in Britain it would be unlikely for a patient to be able to demand to be admitted only to a certain hospital. The Labour Government's document (Department of Health 2004) which makes provision for patients to choose where they receive treatment explicitly excludes psychiatric hospitals.

Wider aspects of advance directives, which cover life or management issues other than medical treatment, may cause a variety of implementation problems.

They are unlikely to be included in legally binding advance directives and many staff are unlikely to want to implement them.

Psychiatrists are not necessarily negative about all aspects of a legally binding advance directive and there has been some acknowledgement of their usefulness in some rare but extremely difficult cases (Atkinson *et al.* 2003b). An example given was the case of someone with anorexia nervosa, who, after previous episodes of treatment, including re-feeding, might write an advance directive refusing force-feeding. Some people believe that even if this leads to death, a supported death in this fashion might be preferable to a different form of suicide, which might otherwise be the outcome.

Other concerns regarding legally binding advance directives include directives which are ambiguous or have unforeseen consequences which lead to outcomes it is clear the person would not have wanted. Changing advance directives usually depends on the capacity to make that decision.

A final concern from both the service user and professional groups is the person who, with no experience of mental illness or psychiatric treatment, makes a legally binding advance directive. Although any advance directive may be suspect in such circumstances, the need to be able to overturn something which may be based on misapprehension, misinformation or other faulty decision-making could be seen as important. In such circumstances it is unlikely that the advance directive would be seen as competent.

The main reason service users want advance directives to be legally binding is to ensure that their wishes are adhered to. If there were greater trust and belief that advance directives would not be overturned or ignored this legal sledgehammer might not be necessary.

Opt-in and opt-out directives

Advance directives can allow the person either to refuse treatment (opt out) or agree to treatment (opt in) or a mixture of both. In the latter case, for example, a person may refuse some medication but agree to take another. For example, they may refuse depot injections but agree to oral medication.

As mentioned previously, opt-in advance directives have been a more common concept in the USA than Britain and may reflect narrower criteria for commitment (in some cases) and a different health care system. Thus people who know they refuse treatment as they become unwell may want to ensure that they are able to receive services, even if they are not detained. This might not be just about treatment for they may want to be protected from their poor judgement or disinhibition when they become ill. Such behaviour (for example, incurring debts, sexual disinhibition, behaviour damaging personal and work relationships) may be harmful to the person but unlikely to lead to detention and compulsory treatment.

Opt-in has, however, recently been introduced in part of Britain. The Mental Health (Care and Treatment) (Scotland) Act 2003 sets out details of 'how the person would wish to be treated for mental disorder' and only then that 'the patient may also refuse particular treatments or categories of treatment for mental disorder' (Scottish Executive 2005). This, however, applies to people who are detained or are to be compulsorily treated.

One question is whether advance acceptance of treatment is the same type of consent as advance refusal of treatment or whether the two types of decision are qualitatively different. Part of the concern will have to do with the relationship of the advance, capacitous decision with the current, incapacitous decision. An advance refusal of treatment is likely to concur with what the person is saying while ill and unable to make a decision. Someone, however, could refuse treatment when well and then want to take it when ill and unable to make a capacitous decision to consent. The treating doctor may then choose to over-ride the advance directive if it were then possible to treat the person under mental health legislation. Some may also choose to treat the patient even if not under compulsory powers on the grounds that it is in the patient's best interests.

An advance agreement to treatment, however, puts the former, capacitous person at odds with the present, non-capable person who is now refusing treatment. This raises complex questions to do with the nature of autonomy and will be dealt with in Chapters 6 and 9.

As compulsory, or mandated, treatment in the community becomes a more common option (Monahan et al. 2001) the possibility of using an opt-in advance directive to avoid compulsory treatment may increase, particularly where the criteria for compulsory treatment in the community are less than for hospital treatment. This raises the possibility of an advance directive being used as one more form of leverage to comply with treatment. Patients may be persuaded that being treated under an opt-in advance directive (and thus being voluntarily treated) is 'better' (e.g. less stigmatising) than being treated involuntarily. The person may feel no less compelled by the opt-in advance directive than by involuntary treatment and, in using the directive, loses any potential safeguards provided by the law.

Medical treatment only or wide ranging content
The end-of-life advance directive, or do-not-resuscitate order, is by its nature a directive regarding medical treatment. Birth plans, however, will cover both medical interventions (such as pain relief) and also a wider range of issues surrounding the birth, from type of music to what happens immediately after the

birth. The difference here is to manage a normal event which is taking place in an environment over which the mother can usually exert little control, and which is geared to the unusual, unexpected, and particularly the hazardous.

Advance directives in mental health sit somewhere between the two. The psychiatric crisis is not wholly unexpected and the person will be trying to manage the 'normal' along with the 'ill'. It is only to be expected that people may want to specify what they want to happen, or not happen, to them as well as treatment. The person may want to specify things they believe will help them recover, including how and when they want to be left alone, exercise, leisure activities, sleeping habits, food, smoking, religious activities and so forth. A comprehensive example is given by Dace (2001).

Some people may want to include much wider aspects of their lives, such as finances, childcare, pet care and security of their home. The more wide ranging the advance directive the more problems there will be putting it into effect. It will not always be clear, for example, who is to be responsible for such aspects. It might be reasonably supposed that childcare will fall under the remit of social workers. They, however, will have to ensure that directions given comply with the Children Act. Who sorts out care of a pet, however, may fall to the most animal-loving member of staff. Taking a patient's credit cards away from them, even if in an advance directive, may not seem an appropriate part of the duties of most clinical staff. In discussions about the remit of advance directives some nurses were very concerned about what might be expected of them, and very clear that they did not want to be responsible for credit cards in such circumstances (Atkinson et al. 2003b).

Scotland has made provision for these issues in some respects by suggesting a two-part statement. The first is the advance statement, which appears in the Act, and the second, a personal statement, which appears in the Guide to Advance Statements (Scottish Executive 2004). This personal statement suggests the person write about their values and reasons for choices so that decisions are made in the light of a wider understanding of the person. Interestingly, this personal statement is not referred to in the Code of Practice (Scottish Executive 2005) thus leaving its position, and indeed knowledge about it, unclear.

Independent or co-operative advance directives
This dimension had largely been dealt with earlier in this chapter, particularly in relation to advance agreements which are made co-operatively with staff. These will be discussed further in Chapter 14. These directives are linked to the last of the dimensions to be covered, that is the intended outcome of advance directives.

The intended outcome of advance directives

The intended outcome of an advance directive is usually taken so much for granted that it is not spelt out in any detail. It is only when this is attempted, whether for research or for other purposes, that it becomes clear that, like so much to do with advance directives, things are not simple and that the philosophies behind them may differ.

The usual statement, that an advance directive is what the person wants when well (capable) to happen when they are ill (incapable), is a statement of purpose or intent. It does not necessarily specify the outcome. Maybe the obvious outcome is 'Does this happen?' Put another way, 'Does the person get what they want?', is a wider question since what the person intended by the advance directive may not be what they achieve when it is put into place.

If, however, advance directives are seen as having a different purpose, that of improving communication between patient and doctor, this will be what is measured as outcome. This purpose will also determine the model of advance directive employed, namely an advance agreement, which forces the two parties to talk together, negotiate and finally agree.

Research studies, however, have looked at some other outcome measures, often related to service use. To make sense of this the advance directive would have to be written with this outcome in mind, and it is not clear that this has always been the case. These issues may be more important to professionals than to the person making the advance directive. Thus the question, 'Whose outcome?' is one of considerable significance.

Advance directives for research

One area of advance planning not usually considered as central to making an advance directive is participation in research when capacity has been either temporarily or permanently lost. Proposals have been made for using advance directives, particularly those involving or limited to appointing a proxy, to allow people with a fluctuating mental illness to take part in research (Backlar 1998; Berg 1996; Bonnie 1997; Dresser 1996; Moorhouse and Weisstub 1996; Shore 2006).

Interest has also been expressed in the potential for advance directives to allow people with dementia to take part in research (Backlar 1998; Keyserling *et al.* 1995; Moorhouse and Weisstub 1996; Sachs 1994; Sachs *et al.* 1994). For people with a permanent incapacity, including dementia, different laws may apply. The Adults with Incapacity (Scotland) Act 2000, for example, makes provision for the inclusion of research for people unable to consent.

Backlar (1998) listed the competencies required to make a research advance directive. These include being able to make the distinction between being a patient and a 'research subject'. An interesting point arises in relation to capacity. Backlar (1998) suggested that although instructions can only be changed when the person has capacity, they should be able to withdraw from research and cancel the advance directive regardless of capacity, and any 'refusal to participate in a research protocol' must be honoured 'at all times' regardless of capacity. This is different from an advance refusal authorising treatment, but is only reasonable since it is a requirement of research protocols that patients be told they can withdraw at any time without giving a reason.

Since most of the discussion on this comes from the USA there is an assumption that the advance directive is actually the appointing of a proxy and thus guidelines are given for the appropriate qualities of a proxy for this type of decision (Backlar 1998). As with other areas of proxy decision-making the proxy should understand the wishes and values of the person for whom they are making a decision. There is some suggestion that particularly for research the concordance between patients and their carers may be poor (Bravo, Paquet and Dubois 2003; Stocking *et al.* 2006).

In some jurisdictions it is only a proxy decision-maker who is considered appropriate to consent to research and a written advance instruction would not be acceptable. The American Psychiatric Association's Task Force on Research Ethics (2006) recommended that: 'States facilitate the use of proxy decision-makers in research involving adults with impaired decisional capacity by authorising the person empowered under state law to make surrogate treatment decisions to also make research decisions...' (p.556).

The Task Force indicated that this power be constrained by the ethical and regulatory boundaries 'analogous to those defined in U.S. federal regulations governing research involving children' (p.556).

Backlar (1998) also gives a list of safeguards which should be legally binding. This includes the patient's doctor having no involvement with the research protocol, and requiring the proxy and patient's doctor to 'work closely together to ensure the subject's welfare'.

One study (Muthappan, Forster and Wendler 2005) of research advance directives found that only 11 per cent of inpatients made them. Of these, 13 per cent were unwilling to participate in research in the future. Of those who were, the majority (76%) would participate in research that would help them and 49 per cent were willing to take part in research which was not of benefit to them, but which had only minimal risk. Only 9 per cent would take part if the risk were more than minimal. Based on these findings the authors concluded that relying on research advance directives 'could block important research' and suggested the need for more flexible approaches. Elsewhere it was noted that although both patients and proxies were willing to discuss participation in a research study at a later date, a 'sizeable minority' did not wish to cede decisions on this to a proxy (Stocking *et al.* 2006).

Advance directives for physical health for people with mental illness

This is a largely unexplored area for people with a mental illness who do not have dementia. It may be something which needs separate consideration from directives covering mental health care. It would be interesting to explore the relationship between the two, and whether having one type of advance directive might predispose towards making the other. Where a mental health advance directive is made under legislation authorising advance directives in general medicine there is no reason why they cannot be combined in one document.

There is an increase in the number of patients with a medical as well as a psychiatric problem in psychiatric hospitals. For example, cases of medical co-morbidity on a general psychiatric ward increased by 14 per cent over three years (Peters and Chiverton 2003) and the number of patients who died of natural causes whilst hospitalised for mental illness increased (Kamara, Peterson and Dennis 1998). On investigation it was shown that two-thirds of those who died had an organic mental disorder.

Staff at one 'chronic psychiatric unit for male veterans', where patients had a mean age of 67.4 years, were surprised to find that 83 per cent (15/18) patients had the capacity to make an advance directive and that of those 80 per cent (12/15) had already completed an advance directive (Valleto *et al.* 2002). More had appointed a health care proxy than had signed a living will. This was not the case everywhere.

Elsewhere one mental health service reported that between one-quarter and one-third of their case-managed clients had a co-morbid medical condition which required medical treatment and follow-up. This resulted in an ambitious programme to develop the use of end-of-life plans for people with severe mental illness as part of their individual service plan (Promoting Excellence undated). Of a group of 142 patients with serious mental illness 27 per cent reported existing preferences for their medical care should they become seriously ill, but only 5 per cent had discussed this with their doctor (Foti *et al.* 2005a). An assessment of patients' responses to hypothetical medical illness scenarios suggested that the majority were able to respond to these difficult questions with only 'moderate distress' (Foti *et al.* 2005b). Although a few terminated the interview, none 're-quired crisis intervention or experienced psychiatric decompensation'. This may reassure those who have concerns about patients with severe mental illness being able to cope with such questions.

There should be no reason to discriminate against people with a mental illness in making an advance directive about their physical health or end-of-life care and some of the competency concerns for mental health advance directives might not apply. The person who lacks insight into their mental condition may be able to make completely competent decisions about end-of-life care. Peters and Chiverton (2003) discuss how nurses might have a useful role in this.

One area of potential concern is people with depression, which may cause them to underestimate their quality of life and health values. This has been demonstrated in surveys of advance directives with both elderly people and carers and suggests that depression may need to be treated before end-of-life advance directives are made.

CHAPTER 5

Advance Directives and the Law

Advance directives in relation to general health care are available in most Western countries, although in some places this may be restricted to advance refusals, or may only apply in specific situations, such as terminal illness or permanent unconsciousness. In most places advance directives for psychiatric care can be made under the general law on advance directives, although in most cases this is implicit, or even assumed if the law is silent on the matter. A growing minority of places have specific legislation regarding advance directives for mental health, or the more general legal provisions have been amended to include a specific section on mental health care. In some cases the law states specifically that the advance directive does not apply if the person is detained under the Mental Health Act. Where the law is a general health advance directive this is less likely to be mentioned specifically, but it would always be assumed that the provisions of a mental health act to detain or compulsorily treat a person 'trump' an advance directive. Only in a minority of cases does the law make specific provision for advance directives to be considered when a person is subject to a mental health act, for example in Scotland. Similarly it is in a minority of cases that mental health advance directives are incorporated into a mental health act.

What is defined in law as an advance directive also varies. Although in some jurisdictions it is assumed to mean a written document stating the person's wishes, in others it includes, or is only the appointment of, a proxy decision-maker. Some jurisdictions allow for an oral statement to serve as an advance directive, but not others. The use of proxies also varies, as does terminology. Thus there are powers of attorney, which may be durable or enduring; an agent may or may not be equivalent to a proxy or power of attorney as might a surrogate. Decisions might be based on best interest or substituted decisions.

The background to the law also varies. Munby (1998) contrasted the position of the interests of the state in the USA and England. Case law in the USA has provided '...four potentially countervailing state interests: 1. the interest of the state in preserving life; 2. the interest of the state in preventing suicide; 3. the interest of the state in maintaining the integrity of the medical profession; and 4. the interest of the state in protecting the innocent third parties' (p.317).

This contrasts with English law, where the first three have never been treated 'as capable of prevailing against the individual's right of self-determination'. Thus self-determination takes priority 'over the sanctity of human life'.

Consent has a long history with its first legal appearance occurring in a British court in 1767 and informed consent not appearing until 1957 in a Californian court case (Mazur 2006). Although clinically the concepts of informed consent and informed refusal of consent are important and probably similar in both countries, there are some legal differences (Munby 1998).

There is no single unifying legal position in relation to advance directives in mental health and, despite their existence in some jurisdictions for some time, there is still little case law, although there is considerable speculation. For these reasons this chapter does not set out to describe individual laws in any detail. Rather it will consider broad positions and the major issues in the inter-relationship between the law and advance directives in mental health care.

For information on the legal position in all the states, territories and provinces of Australia, Canada, the USA and New Zealand, an email survey was carried out between May and July 2006, with some follow-up ongoing until November 2006. Departments of Health/Mental Health were targeted in the first instance. Where replies were not forthcoming, information was pursued via other sources, including voluntary organisations (see Table 5.1).

Most of what has been written about the law and advance directives in mental health has come from the USA, presumably because they have been in existence there for longer than elsewhere and are most prevalent. It does, however, mean that the intricacies of the USA law loom large, and care is needed that they do not overwhelm discussion in other jurisdictions. In the USA, for example, the relationship of the law to the Constitution is paramount; in Europe the emphasis is on the European Directive on Human Rights and national human rights acts.

The main area for consideration is thus the relationship between the law and ethical principles in implementing advance directives. This includes:

- over-riding advance directives

- the right to refuse treatment and the relationship with detention and compulsory treatment under a mental health act

- the right to request treatment

- assessment of capacity.

With all of these there are likely to be some differences between directives which opt in or opt out of treatment. First, however, a brief overview of the international position reveals how complex the scene is.

The international position on advance directives

United Kingdom

Scotland is the only country in the UK which has a specific provision for an advance directive in mental health – in the form of an advance statement – under its Mental Health (Care and Treatment) (Scotland) Act 2003 (Scottish Executive 2003; Scottish Parliament 2003). This provision has two aspects. First, it allows the person to specify both the treatment they do want and the treatment they do not want. Second, it is designed to be taken into consideration when a person is to be treated under the Act. A person can also make an advance statement which outlines wider aspects of care and management, including care of dependants. The law does not allow for a person to appoint a proxy or surrogate decision-maker. A noteworthy dimension of the Scottish law is that the advance statement is designed to come into effect when the person is being compulsorily treated. Both the treating doctor and the tribunal have to take account of it. Although it can be over-ridden this may be the closest the law currently gets to legally enforcing an advance directive.

In England and Wales the government is still trying to reform the Mental Health Act 1983 (Atkinson 2006). A third Bill was put before Parliament in November 2006 (Dyer 2006) and received its first Parliamentary defeat in January 2007 (Dyer 2007).

The lack of specific provision does not mean that an advance directive for mental health cannot be made under common law, which is recognised by the Department of Health (2001a, 2001b) and has led some health authorities to produce their own policies and guidelines (e.g. Derbyshire Mental Health Services NHS Trust 2003, 2004).

Although proxy decision-makers cannot be appointed, it is possible for an advance directive to suggest who the person would like involved in their care, and these people may then be used as a good source of information about the person's preferences and values.

Australia

Each region of Australia (Australian Capital Territory, New South Wales, Northern Territory, Queensland, Victoria and Western Australia) has a separate mental health legislation and policy. In no jurisdiction is there specific legislation enabling mental health advance directives and the position with making mental health advance directives under general law varies. Thus in Victoria a competent person can sign a 'refusal of treatment' certificate or can appoint a Medical Enduring Power of Attorney, who can sign such a certificate on their behalf. Implicitly this would cover mental health. New South Wales, however, only allows for the appointment of a proxy. Western Australia currently has no provision for either written advance directives or the appointment of a proxy but the Acts Amendment (Advance Care Planning) Bill 2006 (currently before Parliament) may have limited application. Elsewhere the Australian Capital Territory (ACT) Mental Health Strategy Action Plan 2003–8 aims to 'establish advance agreements as a routine component of care planning' (cited in Wauchope 2006).

In addition the ACT Legislative Assembly issued a direction, 'Director of Public Prosecutions Direction 2006 No. 2' to continue to protect the rights of patients to make advance refusal of treatment and to protect health professionals from prosecution if death should occur through following such a directive (Stanhope 2006). This was seen as necessary following the enactment of the Commonwealth Euthanasia Laws Act 1997.

The position on advance directives in general, and the regional laws covering them, is discussed by Biegler *et al.* (2000). Knowledge about them is lacking and more research is needed to increase their use (Taylor and Tan 2000).

Canada

The different regions of Canada all have different mental health laws. The position on mental health advance directives also differs and is not usually dealt with under the Mental Health Act. In Ontario, for example, they are covered in the Ontario Substitute Decisions Act 1992 which allows for a power of attorney for personal care. Gray, Shone and Liddle (in press) describe this as 'a good example of how advance directive legislation can be used to establish a Ulysses contract for psychiatric treatment'. The Act allows for the person making the advance directive (the grantor) to state the circumstances of the advance directive being triggered, including assessment by a non-official person, or a second situation where an assessment is made by an official assessor.

In British Columbia the Representation Agreement Act 1996 allows for 'representation agreement' for an opt-in to treatment (or Ulysses contract) and also for opt-out provision with the specific condition that a person cannot refuse involuntary admission or care and treatment while an involuntary patient either in hospital or on leave in the community. A similar provision is in the British Columbia Health Care (Consent) and Facilities (Admission) Act 1996. Thus the provisions of the Mental Health Act are upheld (Gray *et al.*, in press).

The different regional laws also make different provisions for assessment of capacity before making an advance directive. Thus the Manitoba Mental Health Act and the Nova Scotia Involuntary Psychiatric Treatment Act 2005 do not require capacity tests before making an advance directive, but do allow for an over-ride if honouring the advance directive would harm either the involuntary patient or another person, in which case the 'best interests' criterion is applied. Even within one region different laws may not be congruent. Thus in Ontario the Substitute Decisions Act requires the person to be assessed by a professional assessor as to their capacity, and to have their advance directive witnessed when making certain 'serious' provisions, whereas the Health Care Consent Act does not. This, however, requires the advance directive to be applicable in the current circumstances, and can thus be over-ruled if it does not meet this when the best interest test is used.

New Zealand
Although there is no specific law in New Zealand to allow mental health advance directives, all advance directives (general and psychiatric) are allowed under common law and are implicit in the New Zealand Bill of Rights Act 1990. It is possible to appoint a proxy. Enduring powers of attorney for welfare and for property can be appointed under separate legislation.

In respect of the need for capacity to change an advance directive this has not been tested in the courts but a respondent from the Mental Health Commission suggested that 'revocation would likely be challenged if competence was in doubt' (see www.mhc.govt.nz/advance).

The World Health Organisation (2005) described the issues in making an advance directive in New Zealand and examples of how it might be used.

United States of America
The legal position on advance directives in the USA must be set against the background of the Patient Self-Determination Act 1990 (passed as part of the Omnibus Budget Reconciliation Act) which is a federal statute covering all states and came into effect in December 1991. It provides for patients to make an advance directive either as a written document or by appointing a durable power of attorney for health care. It only applies to service providers who receive Medicare and Medicaid funding from the government to cover all patients treated in or through such service providers. Amongst the requirements of the law are that the service providers must have written policies and follow certain procedures in respect of advance directives; the patient's medical record must indicate whether or not an advance directive exists; service providers do not discriminate against an individual based on whether or not there is an advance directive; service providers provide information for the patient about how to make a complaint about the use of their advance directive and provide education for staff, patients and the community about advance directives (Dunlap 2000–1; Emanuel 2004; Greco et al. 1991).

This law allows patients with a mental illness to execute an advance directive in respect of both their general health and end-of-life situations, and also their mental health care, although this may be modified by state statute. In many cases this can be achieved in one document and with one agent, although separate advance directives and agents are also permissible and some might find them preferable.

The fact that hospitals and nursing homes must provide information on making an advance directive at the time of hospital admission (or earlier in respect of some situations) may not be appropriate for patients entering a psychiatric hospital who may be at the least confused, if not incompetent, at the time and thus unable to take advantage of such a provision.

The provisions of this law across the USA vary. In Alabama, for example, not only is there no provision for mental health advance directives, but advance directives only exist for end-of-life situations and pain relief. Some states have full provision for written psychiatric advance directives (PADs) and the appointment of a proxy or power of attorney, although some require both to be in place. Some states only allow for the appointment of a proxy or power of attorney and not for a written advance directive. Provisions of the law for each of the 50 states are provided in Table 5.1. The information is derived from the formerly mentioned survey, state-based web sources, and the National Resource Centre on Psychiatric Advance Directives and was compiled in the summer of 2006.

Looking at individual provisions in the law relating to mental health care the majority of states allow the appointment of a health care agent to make some decisions about mental health care (49 out of 50 states); to write a separate legal advance instruction (46/50); to consent to medication or specify medication (46/50); and to refuse medication (44/50). Just over three-quarters (39/50) of states allow consent or preferences as to hospitalisation; and two-thirds (33/50) refusal of hospitalisation. One-third (18/50) only allow advance instructions to be written on the form appointing a health care agent. Three states require a court determination of legal incompetence before an advance directive can be invoked. Only two states require both an advance instruction and a health care agent: that competence to write the PAD is certified by a qualified mental health professional and that a mental health professional must agree the appropriateness of the provisions laid out in the PAD (National Resource Centre on Psychiatric Advance Directives 2006).

Table 5.1. Provisions of the law relating to advance directives for each state in the USA

	Specific law/provision			General law				Comments
	Written PAD	Proxy/ DPA only	Both/ either	Written	Proxy/ DPA only	Both/ either	Explicit/ implicit	
Alabama	No	No	–	No	No	–	–	Advance directive only allows for end-of-life and pain relief
Alaska	Yes	–	Yes	–	–	–	–	–
Arizona	No	Yes	–	–	–	–	–	–
Arkansas	No	No	–	No	Yes	–	Explicit	–
California	No	No	–	In part	In part	–	–	Some aspects of medical health care explicitly excluded
Colorado	No	No	–	No	Yes	–	Implicit	–
Connecticut	No	No	–	–	–	Yes	–	Check internet
Delaware	No	No	–	–	–	Yes	Implicit	–
Florida	No	No	–	–	–	Yes	Implicit	Advance directives made in other states are valid
Georgia	No	No	–	No	Yes	–	Implicit	–
Hawaii	Yes	–	Yes	–	–	–	–	–
Idaho	Yes	–	Yes	–	–	–	–	–

State							Notes
Illinois	Yes	—	Yes	—	—	—	—
Indiana	Yes	—	Yes	—	—	—	PADs are embedded in the general law
Iowa	No	No	—	No	Yes	Implicit	—
Kansas	No	No	—	No	Yes	Implicit	—
Kentucky	Yes	—	Yes	—	—	—	Amendment to, and embedded in, general law
Louisiana	Yes	Yes	—	—	—	—	Check embedded in general law or mental health law?
Maine	Yes	—	Yes	—	—	—	Specific section of general law?
Maryland	Yes	—	Yes	—	—	—	Check embedded general law?
Massachusetts	No	No	—	No	Yes	Implicit	—
Michigan	No	Yes	—	—	—	—	Embedded in general law
Minnesota	Yes	—	Yes	—	—	—	—
Mississippi	—	—	—	Yes	Yes	Implicit	—
Missouri	No	—	No	No	Yes	Implicit	—
Montana	Yes	—	Yes	—	—	—	—

Continued on next page

Table 5.1 continued

	Specific law/provision			General law				Comments
	Written PAD	Proxy/DPA only	Both/either	Written	Proxy/DPA only	Both either	Explixit/implicit	
Nebraska	No	No	–	No	Yes	–	–	–
Nevada	No	No	–	No	Yes	–	Implicit	–
New Hampshire	No	No	–	No	Yes	–	Implicit	–
New Jersey	Yes	–	Yes	–	–	–	–	–
New Mexico	Yes	–	Yes	–	–	–	–	–
New York	No	–	No	No	Yes	–	Implicit	–
North Carolina	Yes	–	Yes	–	–	–	–	–
North Dakota	No	No	–	Yes	–	Yes	Implicit	–
Ohio	Yes	–	Yes	–	–	–	–	–
Oklahoma	Yes	–	Yes	–	–	–	–	–
Oregon	Yes	–	Yes	–	–	–	–	–
Pennsylvania	Yes	–	Yes	–	–	–	–	Embedded in general law
Rhode Island	No	–	No	No	Yes	–	Implicit	–

South Carolina	No	No	—	No	Yes	Implicit	—
South Dakota	Yes	—	Yes	—	—	—	—
Tennessee	Yes	—	Yes	—	—	—	—
Texas	Yes	—	Yes	—	—	—	—
Utah	Yes	—	Yes	—	—	—	—
Vermont	No	No	—	No	Yes	Implicit	—
Virginia	No	No	—	No	Yes	Implicit	—
Washington	Yes	—	Yes	—	—	—	—
West Virginia	No	No	—	No	Yes	Implicit	—
Wisconsin	No	No	—	No*	Yes	Implicit	Specific exclusions relating to mental health care re. proxy.
Wyoming	Yes	—	Yes	—	—	—	—

* A response from the Bureau of Mental Health and Substance Abuse Service arrived in answer to the question: 'Is it possible to make a psychiatric advance directive under legislation to make a general health care directive?'

It is possible to add additional information to either a living will or a durable power of attorney for health care to clarify what the intents and wishes of the principal are. This is implicit in the state statutes.

Florida, which implicitly allows for a mental health advance directive in its statute, Chapter 765 Health Care Advance Directives, has a wide-ranging definition of advance directives as meaning 'a witnessed written document or oral statement…and includes, but is not limited to, the designation of a health care surrogate, a living will, or an anatomical gift'. The law also makes the following special provision: 'an advance directive executed in another state in compliance with the law of that state or of this state is validly executed for the purpose of this chapter' (765.112).

California puts restrictions on what another person may consent to on behalf of a patient, specifically excluding 'commitment to a placement in mental health treatment facility', 'convulsive treatment' and psychosurgery (along with sterilisation and abortion) (California Codes, Probate Code Health Care Decisions Law, Section 46.52). To this Wisconsin adds 'experimental mental health research' and 'drastic mental health treatment procedures'. Other restrictions may cover the length or time in hospital or a treatment facility. Idaho, for example, in its definition of mental health treatment includes 'short-term admission to a treatment facility for a period not to exceed seventeen days' (Title 66.601 (5)).

The standard for capacity to make an advance directive varies from requiring the person to be of sound mind to a formal assessment by a psychiatrist or psychologist (Srebnik and Kim 2006).

In states which do not recognise non-married partners, appointing a partner as a health care agent gives them legal rights and responsibilities and has been used in some states to promote advance directives (e.g. Michigan) (Potts 2005). In Maryland an update to the general advance directive in 2006 by extending the rights of the appointed proxy was promoted as giving same sex partners rights if they were appointed as health care agents (Lynsen 2006). This should be true elsewhere where same sex partners may otherwise lack status.

The Protection and Advocacy for Individuals with Mental Illness (PAIMI) programme (www.mentalhealth.samhsa.gov/cmhs/PAIMI) has information on the application of the law in each state. The programme is working to maximise the effectiveness of advance directives as a tool for self-determination (Priaulx 2003) and its web site gives details of its activities in each state.

A web site recently set up by Duke University gives information on psychiatric advance directives in the USA (http://pad.duhs.duke.edu/background.htm). The Bazelon Centre for Mental Health Law also has information on the legal position, with details on New York, North Carolina, Nebraska and Washington DC and discussion about Vermont and Washington (www.bazelon.org/).

Over-riding advance directives

Some mental health service users are clear that advance directives should be legally enforceable and that clinicians should not have the power to over-ride them. Without this, they would argue, an advance directive is worthless. Since the power to over-ride them exists in some form in all jurisdictions this might be seen as limiting both their acceptance (or willingness to make one) and their usefulness. Indeed some laws, such as those in North Carolina, include a list of conditions which allow the advance directive to be over-ridden which are 'so broad that it is unlikely that a physician or other mental health provider will ever feel compelled to honour an advance directive if he or she is not otherwise inclined to do so' (Bazelon Centre for Mental Health Law undated). How reasonable is it that clinicians can over-ride an advance directive? The response will tend to depend on the justification for the reasons given.

Brock (1991) described three situations in which a physician might over-ride an advance directive in physical health care. These were:

- where good reasons exist to question whether the advance directive is an accurate, that is current, reflection of the person's wishes

- where the advance directive conflicts with the present interests or 'personal identity' of the person

- where the interests of others need to take precedence.

This was developed by Swanson et al. (2006a), looking specifically at mental health advance directives. They noted that although people who have recurrent crises or acute episodes of a serious mental illness may also have considerable experience of past treatment, including emergency treatment, this does not necessarily mean that their advance directive will be adhered to. In Washington DC, however, there is an expectation that the treatment preferences of a consumer will be followed except for 'good cause' and 'shall never be over-ridden for the convenience of the Department or other provider'.

Some decisions to over-ride an advance directive may come from the treating doctor's own ethical position and different policies/laws will reflect differently on this. The Department of Health (2001b), for example, states that: 'A health professional may not over-ride a valid and applicable advance refusal on the grounds of the professional's personal conscientious objections to such a refusal' (p.11). In some cases this may require the treating doctor to hand care over to someone who can support the provisions of the advance directive.

In response to a vignette, 47 per cent of psychiatrists in North Carolina indicated that they would over-ride a psychiatric advance directive, even if known to be valid and competently made, where it refused hospitalisation and medication. Factors which contributed to this were working in an emergency department, having concern about the patient's violence and lack of insight, and being 'legally defensive' (Swanson *et al.* 2007).

Reasons for over-riding advance directives will differ, in some instances, depending on whether they are opt-in or opt-out directives. For opt-out or treatment refusal, reasons given include the following:

- leaving the patient untreated is not in their best interests because:

  - they may spend a longer time in hospital

  - a long period of illness will hinder recovery (either to mental state, personal or social life or employment)

  - they may actively harm themselves

  - they may die

- leaving the patient untreated is not in the best interests of others because:

  - long periods in hospital (when the patient *could* be treated) are unacceptable

- drain on resources

  - patients who are acutely ill are difficult to nurse and distressing to other patients

  - for patients who are dangerous it is an unacceptable risk for staff and other patients.

Where the advance directive is an opt-in to treatment reasons will include the following:

- the treatment is inappropriate (e.g. contra-indications for a particular drug, contravenes clinical good practice guidelines)

- the clinician still wants a second opinion (e.g. for electro-convulsive therapy (ECT))

- resource issues/funding is not available because:

  - the service is outwith the catchment/referral area

  - private insurance or the National Health Service (NHS) will not pay for the particular intervention/drug

- the service is inappropriate (e.g. entry criteria are not met by the patient)

- the service/resource has a long waiting list (or similar) and the advance directive would result in inappropriate/unfair preferential treatment (leading to a two-tier system)

- the service/resource does not exist.

Some reasons have to do with the advance directive itself:

- it is not clear the person had capacity when it was made

- it is not clear the person was fully informed of choices

- it is not clear the person was fully informed of consequences

- the instructions are unclear

- the advance directive is 'old'/out-of-date/has not been reviewed recently

- the advance directive does not conform to local statute/requirements, e.g. not properly witnessed.

In discussion with service users, Atkinson *et al.* (2003a) found that a number had not thought through the consequences of their treatment choices, especially in relation to treatment refusal. If this became apparent at a later stage it would seem to give clinicians a legitimate reason for over-riding an advance directive. It also points to the advantage of having a professional involved in drawing up the advance directive, or at least discussing it with the patient so that their choice is fully informed.

Different laws make provision for doctors (or others) to over-ride advance directives. Thus in Scotland there are requirements to inform the Mental Welfare Commission as well as the patient, and the decision to over-ride the advance statement can be upheld by the tribunal. One study in the USA, however, indicated that 62 per cent of patients with schizophrenia or a related condition supported the view that doctors should pay a legal penalty for not following an advance directive compared with 38 per cent of family members and only 11 per cent of clinicians (Swanson *et al.* 2003).

In Pennsylvania the law specifies circumstances under which a 'physician or other mental health care provider cannot in good conscience comply' which includes 'the instructions are contrary to good clinical practice', 'the treatment is unavailable' or 'if the policies of a mental health care provider preclude compliance'. The latter provision may include, for example, a requirement not to drink alcohol. There is a provision that in such circumstances the physician or provider 'shall make every reasonable effort to assist in the transfer of the declarant or principle to another physician or mental health provider who will comply with the declaration...' (Pennsylvania Consolidate Statutes Title 20 Descendants, Estates and Fiduciaries Chapter 58 Mental Health Care 5804).

It may be that the 'immunity' clause in some legislation, which allows a clinician to over-ride an advance directive and treat a patient, is being 'misconstrued' (Szmukler and Dawson 2006). They argued that a clinician could only treat a patient with an advance refusal if they had 'clear legal power to do so' through civil commitment.

One way of ignoring an advance directive, but without being seen to over-ride it overtly, is for the service provider/clinician to refuse to declare the person incompetent and thus the advance directive is not invoked (Priaulx 2003).

Taking a somewhat broader approach Bernstein (2006) suggested that the main problem was the mental health system itself, quoting the (USA) President's New Freedom Commission on Mental Health, that the system is 'in shambles'. His argument was that by 'myopically' concentrating on 'immediate crises' the mental health services perpetuate the problems they are supposed to alleviate. Thus the practical (and possibly legal) approach taken to advance directives 'cannot be disaggregated from these legal realities'. Furthermore he argued that it is failures in the mental health service itself which cause people to have crises and that if this were addressed there would be no need to activate advance directives.

It is not just mental health advance directives which are over-ridden and care should be taken not to assume that it is only a reflection of mental health services or attitudes to psychiatric patients. Most research in this area has considered – maybe not surprisingly – end-of-life directives. A study of intended compliance with a do-not-resuscitate (DNR) order based on a case scenario indicated that one-third of German doctors would not comply with the DNR in respect of cardiopulmonary resuscitation. This was in contrast with 8 per cent of Swedish nurses' responses to the same scenario (Richter and Eisemann 1999). In another study in Italy 58 per cent of physicians in intensive care units (ICUs) (total sample 225) indicated 'they would not respect the expressed desire of a patient to forego treatment' (Giannini, Pessina and Tacchi 2003).

A more positive finding came from Finnish physicians (Hildén, Louhiala and Palo 2004) where 92 per cent (of 432) had a positive attitude towards living wills and 86 per cent endorsed totally or partially the statement, 'By the time the living will is needed it should be unconditionally respected'. Only 2 per cent of respondents had a particularly negative attitude to living wills. A small majority (55%) had not been involved in using a living will.

Nevertheless, the Bazelon Centre for Mental Health Law (undated) 'urge as the guiding principle for state law and policy that psychiatric advance directives operate in exactly the same way as any other advance directive, subject, if at all, only to narrowly drawn and legitimate emergency situations'.

The right to refuse treatment and mental health legislation

A competent adult has the right to refuse treatment for, as Lord Templeman put it, 'reasons which are rational, irrational or for no reason' (cited in Munby 1998, p.316). To treat someone without their consent would leave the treating doctor open to a charge of battery or assault or similar, although the law recognises special cases of emergency treatment where the person is unable to consent. In such cases it is assumed that treatment is in the person's best interests. An advance directive (refusal) will make the person's wishes clear if they are unable to state them because of temporary, or now permanent, incapacity.

This right to refuse treatment is firmly based on the ethical principle of autonomy and the person's right to determine what happens to their body. It is a right which has received more recognition in the courts than in legislation, but advance statutes are a way of enshrining this right (Cerminara 2003). In the USA the United States Supreme Court recognised the refusal of treatment as a fundamental right. It has been argued that in using an opt-in directive a person essentially waives that right, and that there are conditions put upon this waiver (Anderson 2003). Anderson suggested that not all advance directive laws, specifically in this case Washington's, sufficiently safeguard this right to refusal. It is made, he argued, sufficiently clear to patients that the advance directive is irrevocable, and that they may, therefore, at some point be treated, even though at the time they refuse (if judged incompetent).

There may be some limitation placed on what can be refused, for example many services do not allow a person to refuse pain relief or palliative care, nutrition and hydration or general nursing care to maintain hygiene. Even here there may be exceptions. Pain relief can be refused in birth plans and may also be deemed acceptable as unwanted for practitioners of certain religions such as Buddhism or Hinduism. It is also noted in some guidelines that 'some patients may prefer to tolerate levels of discomfort if this means they remain able to communicate with family, friends etc.' (Derbyshire Mental Health Services NHS Trust 2003).

Derbyshire Mental Health Services NHS Trust (2003) gives clear advice to clinicians that: 'A valid verbal or written advance directive refusing food, i.e. one made by a person who knows that this refusal will lead to death, should be followed and the person cannot be force fed or fed artificially when they become incompetent'.

Although an advance refusal which hastens death by refusing life-prolonging treatment is generally accepted (and not treated as suicide) this is different from requests for active euthanasia which are less commonly accepted.

In mental illness, however, the position is not straightforward. Although the principle remains the same, that a capacitous person can refuse treatment, a mental health act is likely to modify this in various ways. Arguments for allowing treatment without consent are discussed elsewhere (Fennell 1996).

The law usually allows for a person to be detained or compulsorily treated because they pose a risk either to themselves or others. This can be determined either more or less narrowly. Thus where the law is narrow this might be best seen as a 'dangerousness' criteria, the danger being to other people, and the risk to self may need to be immediate and severe, such as imminent risk of suicide. Elsewhere the law may allow for a wider definition of risk, including to the person's general health and welfare.

Yet another question arises here. Should people who pose a risk to others be treated differently from those who are a risk to themselves? Philosophers such as John Stuart Mill would argue yes, and that harm to others is the only reason for infringing a person's autonomy. Further questions arise, however. Should a person who has committed a violent act against another (which may not necessarily go through the courts) and who is ill be treated against their wishes? Other violent criminals are not involuntarily 'treated' even where an intervention programme might be available. Co-operation with such may, however, hasten parole. What if the 'patient' is only suspected of being violent? The newer, preventative type of outpatient compulsory treatment orders fit this. There is not the space here to debate these issues and they have been well covered elsewhere (Monahan *et al.* 2001).

Seeking to prevent someone committing a violent act against another person may be seen to be in the best interest of all parties: the person committing the act, the person acted against and society. In terms of advance directives, rather than the function of mental health legislation in general, the issue is not whether the person should be detained, but whether they can or should be detained without being treated. The pragmatic answer for many will be no, for the reason given above: difficulty in managing the person, safety of staff and others, and cost.

A legal position is given by Winick (1997): 'Just as a will provision that violated public policy would be unenforceable, a mental health advance directive seeking to refuse hospitalisation or treatment that would be required to prevent harm to others would be seen as unfeasible' (p.394).

Appelbaum (2006) argued that the mix of *parens patriae* and police powers which underpins all mental health legislation suggests that civil commitment will, and should always, trump an advance refusal of treatment. He concluded: 'That the patient has previously requested that she be allowed to endanger her well-being while under the influence of mental disorder may simply not be material to the state's interest in preventing harm' (p.396).

Another argument might be that those who have committed a crime have given up their right to choose how they are treated. This would justify people not being able to opt out of detention. Treatment, however, is not punishment, nor should it be used as such. There is also the issue that many patients are being detained because of the *risk* of dangerousness (or harm), rather than for something they have done. The concept of preventative detention has been extended in some jurisdictions in recent years and arguments both for and against this have been reviewed.

The law in different jurisdictions varies as to whether a person detained under a mental health act automatically loses the right to refuse treatment. In some, such as Scotland, there is the possibility for a person to be detained but for an advance directive refusing (certain forms of) treatment still being honoured.

In the USA the case of Nancy Hargrave caused some concern (Appelbaum 2004). Ms Hargrave, who had a diagnosis of paranoid schizophrenia and multiple hospital admissions, made an advance directive (which in Vermont, the state in which she lived, was in the form of a durable power of attorney) in which she refused 'any and all antipsychotic, neuroleptic, psychotropic or psychoactive medications'. Before this was used her lawyers, on her behalf and on behalf of all those patients in a similar situation, filed a suit to prevent the state from overriding this during a period of involuntary commitment. At the time Act 114, passed the previous year, allowed hospital (or prison) staff to apply to a court to over-ride such an advance directive, once the directive had stood for 45 days.

The legal challenge was based on the Americans with Disabilities Act (ADA) and the claim that this discriminated against people with a mental disorder under Title II. This provided for the provision of public services, benefits and so forth to be available to all and not excluded by reason of disability. The argument presented was that she was being excluded from exercising the state's durable power of attorney for health care.

Both the District Court and the Second Circuit Court (covering both Vermont and New York) found that Act 114 violated the ADA and thus advance directives cover involuntary as well as voluntary patients. Thus Appelbaum (2004) concluded that: 'Advance directives may now constitute an ironclad bulwark against future involuntary treatment with medication – except in emergencies – even for incompetent, committed patients and even when the alternative is long-term institutional care' (p.763).

This, he pointed out, increases concern, raised by others (Halpern and Szmukler 1997) of psychiatric hospitals filling with untreated patients who cannot be discharged. This fear of clinicians might work against the implementation of advance directives since there is growing evidence for clinicians' involvement in patients completing them. The issue of detention is different and nowhere can anyone opt out of being sectioned. The question of the appropriateness of detention to protect someone against the harm they may cause themselves is outwith the scope of this book.

The question of capacity and mental health legislation is an interesting one in that not all legislation requires the person to be incapacitated before they are compulsorily treated, e.g. the Mental Health Act 1983 in England and Wales. This position has been challenged (Doyal and Sheather 2005). This was the position in Scotland under the Mental Health (Scotland) Act 1984 but was modified in the Mental Health (Care and Treatment) (Scotland) Act 2003, which introduced a criterion of impaired ability to make medical decisions. Since in both countries there is also incapacity legislation the position is, on occasion, somewhat confused. This anomaly, plus the potential problems of having both mental health and incapacity Acts, has led to some questioning whether there should be one legislation covering both (Dawson and Szmukler 2006).

Where the law allows for a capacitous person to be treated against their wishes then it is not unreasonable (within the philosophical framework of such a law) that an advance directive should be over-ridden, irrespective of the criteria for compulsory treatment. Again a discussion of the appropriateness of criteria for compulsory treatment (or compulsorily treating a capacitous person) is outwith the scope of this book.

The right to request treatment

There are two aspects to requesting treatment. One is an advance directive which lays down how the person wants to be treated, for example which medication they want to be treated with and at what dose. The second is a more general opting into treatment, where the person makes it clear they want to be treated, even if at the time they are refusing treatment. As a corollary to this the advance directive may set out what such treatment should be, or may simply state that the patient will abide by their doctor's decision. These advance directives may be extremely detailed, for example that given by Dace (2001).

Nowhere does the law allow a person to demand a specific intervention or medication. The right to consent to treatment is actually 'a power to consent, not a power to compel' (Munby 1998). It is usually suggested that the reasons for this are self-evident. Doctors cannot be compelled to provide treatment which they do not believe to be appropriate or in patients' best interests. This would include treatment not meeting current guidelines for the patient's condition or treatment otherwise contra-indicated for the patient. Treatment where there is no evidence of efficacy may prove difficult for some doctors to agree to, although they may do so if there is no evidence that it causes harm. Such treatments may include the use of megavitamins, other dietary supplements, or homeopathic or herbal medicines. Dace (2001), for example, requested being encouraged to take 'Bach's Rescue Remedy, Bach's Agrimony, and homeopathic arnica and aconite tablets', before trying other treatments.

The assumption here is that it is only the doctor who understands things such as medication and can make appropriate decisions. This overlooks the patient's past experience with different treatments and the impact these have had on them, including emergency treatment. The patient's cost–benefit analysis of particular treatments may vary considerably between doctors (e.g. Chadwick 1997). This is because patients will place a personal value or cost on different aspects of treatment in line with their personal goals and outcomes which may differ from the outcomes seen as important by professionals. To this end many laws allow patients to specify what treatments they want, or what they are prepared to accept, on the understanding that this is provided as a guideline only to the doctor, and can be over-ridden.

Where a patient goes to court to request a particular treatment and the court disagrees with the doctor, the most usual solution would be to find a doctor who supports the court's (and patient's) view rather than coerce the patient's existing doctor (Munby 1998). Policy positions have, however, been challenged in recent years, resulting in trusts being required to provide treatment. One example would be that of Herceptin, which became universally available, regardless of local or other budget implications, as the result of a court case (Barrett *et al.* 2006).

Giving reasons why choices have been made may help a doctor either comply with the request, or, if unable to do so, make a treatment decision which has broadly the same aims. Thus Dace (2001) says: 'When distressed, I am extremely sensitive to noise. I require a quiet, calm environment in which to recompose myself. If I am placed in a noisy environment with excitable people I will become mute, withdrawn and rapidly institutionalised' (p.30).

Other reasons for over-riding advance directive requests have been covered earlier.

The main anxiety for many people about what might be termed a general opt-in advance directive, where someone indicates they are to be treated in the face of contemporaneous refusal, is that this is in the nature of a self-imposed treatment order and similar to what might be posed under a mental health act (Swanson *et al.* 2000). In practical terms this will only become an issue where the person has to be capable before they are able to revoke their advance directive. In some jurisdictions this is referred to as a Ulysses contract. One study suggested that patients were 'less enthusiastic about this form of advance directive, wanting to maintain the option of changing their mind in a crisis' (Swartz *et al.* 2006). This was particularly true for patients with schizophrenia and for non-white (mainly African-American) patients.

The main concern, for both staff treating the patient and for ethicists, is how to resolve the conflict between the competing treatment decisions made by a capable person in the past and a less than competent (but possibly not incapable) person in the present (Dresser 1984; Rhoden 1982; Swanson *et al.* 2006a). The question of which is the 'real choice' or 'authentic voice' of the person is raised, and can lead to challenges about the notion of persons and personhood (see Chapter 7).

Assessment of capacity

A brief note is required here on the terms 'capacity' and 'competence'. Frequently used interchangeably, they are in fact different. There is a need to distinguish between a clinical assessment of mental ability to make specific decisions and a legal determination of the same. Unhelpfully different legal jurisdictions use both incapacity and incompetence as the legal term. In its *Resource Book on Mental Health, Human Rights and Legislation* the World Health Organisation (2005) uses 'capacity' as a health concept and 'competence' as a legal concept (which is the position in the USA). In Britain this is generally reversed.

In all legal jurisdictions there is a presumption in favour of capacity/competence, and incapacity/incompetence has to be demonstrated to the satisfaction of the court. There are three areas where an assessment of capacity will have legal importance in relation to an advance directive: making the advance directive, invoking the advance directive, and revoking the advance directive.

Most jurisdictions specifically require that the person making the advance directive is capable so to do. Where this is not specified, or not witnessed, there will generally be a requirement to demonstrate that the person was capable at the time before it is upheld (particularly where it refuses treatment).

There is a general assumption that the advance directive is invoked when the person has lost capacity. The most variation comes in whether the person has to have capacity to revoke it, although some jurisdictions are specific that the person has to be capable. This is witnessed in the same way as making one (e.g. Scotland). In other places this is not the case.

It is rare for any particular test of capacity, or set of criteria, to be laid out, unless this is part of a capacity/incapacity Act. This can cause some problems in understanding how the capacity is to be assessed and by whom, for in many cases the person who witnesses an advance statement is not witnessing that the person is capable, or at least not by any formal test. Indeed a number of the people specified in different laws as being able to witness advance statements may not have any formal training in the assessment of capacity.

The main features of determining capacity are the person's ability to understand, retain and weigh up information in order to make a choice and then to be able to communicate that choice. A discussion of capacity is outwith the scope of this book but a good, selective review is given by Wong *et al.* (1999).

Much has been written about the assessment of capacity with the seminal work coming from the MacArthur Treatment Competence Study spearheaded by Grisso and Appelbaum (Grisso and Appelbaum 1995, 1996; Grisso *et al.* 1995). An important development in the assessment of capacity is the agreement that capacity is not an all-or-nothing trait, but a function, which a person may move in and out of, or may have for some areas of decision-making but not for others. This is made explicit in the Mental Health (Care and Treatment) (Scotland) Act 2003 where the impaired ability criterion required to subject someone to the Act only refers to their ability to make medical decisions.

One important variable which has particular relevance to the concept of lack of insight is whether the person can make a decision which applies to themself. Thus a person may come to a rational decision about the use of psychotropic medication but still not be able to apply it to themself because they do not believe they are ill. Loss of insight is a medical construct used in diagnosis and should not be confused with, or equated with, loss of capacity or legal incapacity. Some clinicians have argued that lack of insight should form part of a competence test. Thus Van Staden and Krüger (2003) asserted 'that the patient's *acceptance* of the need for a medical intervention should *not* be prevented by his/her mental disorder, is a condition *necessary* for informed consent' (p.42).

To support this they argued that a choice made in such circumstances is not the autonomous choice of the patient but a choice determined by the illness. Such an approach has even led to psychiatrists arguing that 'compulsory treatment should be seen as a form of liberation' (Turner 2004).

Appelbaum and Redlich (2006) found no strong or consistent association between a person's capacity to make decisions (as measured by the MacArthur Competence Assessment Tool, MacCAT) and the use of four different types of 'leverage' (criminal justice system, mental health/civil justice system and social welfare [both housing and benefits]) to 'encourage' adherence to treatment. A note of caution was that the capacity was measured at the time of the study and leverage was an over-time measurement. The authors questioned, nevertheless, widespread practices and assumptions about decisional capacity.

Lack of insight is, however, likely to be used by treating clinicians as a reason for overturning an advance directive which refuses treatment based on a belief of the person that they are not ill. Since approximately one-third of patients with schizophrenia appear to lack insight (Amador *et al.* 1994) this is a substantial minority of patients. On the one hand, patients who do not believe they are ill might be less likely to choose to make an advance directive, reasoning that they are not ill. On the other hand, if they have experienced coercive treatment they might be more inclined to make an advance directive to avoid future treatment. It is in these cases that the standing of the advance directive under the Mental Health Act will be of significance.

The relationship between lack of insight, lack of capacity or competence and mental health law is likely to be fraught with complications unless clear guidance is given, either in the law, or the code of practice regarding this. In New York, for example, the Mental Hygiene Law makes provision for involuntary care and treatment for those who have 'a mental illness for which care and treatment as a patient in a hospital is essential to such person's welfare and whose judgement is so impaired that he is unable to understand the need for such care and treatment' (quoted in Stavis 1993).

It is not only insight that needs to be considered as a 'special case' in relation to competence. The particular consequences of depressive thinking (Rudnick 2002) and anorexia nervosa (Tan, Hope and Stewart 2003) also offer challenges to an assessment of capacity. Treatment for depression, for example, has been shown to have a significant impact on elderly patients' desires to have life-saving treatment (Hooper *et al.* 1996). Appelbaum *et al.* (1999), however, found that out-patients with major depression showed few impairments in their ability to make decisions related to research.

Since capacity is function-specific it should be considered in the context of the specific decision to be taken. This lack of insight about the *need* for treatment does not necessarily mean the person lacks ability to make competent decisions about which treatment they are compelled to take, for example with respect to limiting certain side-effects. This might be expressed at the time or in an advance directive.

PART II

Ideological Issues in Advance Directives

CHAPTER 6

Autonomy and Advance Directives

Respect for the patient is at the heart of medical ethics. The cornerstone of this respect is preservation of the patient's autonomy. Autonomy is thus accepted as the guiding principle, a state to be preserved or a goal for patients to regain. Most commonly autonomy is presented as protecting and respecting the wishes of the patient in relation to the treatment they receive, considered conceptually as the principle of informed consent. Mental health legislation over-rides this principle and, under certain circumstances, allows for the compulsory treatment of patients. It is usually accepted that the patient's autonomy is not really being compromised since, at that particular time, the patient has lost their autonomy as a result of the interference of their mental illness on their actions.

Advance directives require the person making them not only to be capacitous but also to have autonomy – that is, to be making their decision(s) freely and without coercion or undue influence from others. Although, however, autonomy requires capacity, capacity does not ensure autonomy. One problem with linking capacity to autonomy is that the decisions of non-autonomous individuals can be disregarded. Non-capacitous individuals, however, do still have (in many cases) clear preferences and seek to make choices. The difficult question then becomes when are the choices or preferences of non-capacitous individuals to be adhered to and why?

If the major concern of advance directives is consent to, or refusal of, treatment, then paternalism presents a problem, and the debate is between the merits and demerits of each in providing care and treatment to various groups of patients (Häyry 1991). Autonomy needs to be considered in a wider context if it is to be understood in relation to mental illness, mental health law and, in particular, advance directives.

Making an advance directive is about the exercise of autonomy – the autonomy of the capacitous person to decide their treatment in accordance with the principle of informed consent. This may be exercised in different ways. Opting out of the treatment may be motivated by the desire of the well person to preserve more of the autonomy by avoiding the side-effects of some treatments and by accepting periods of their illness as the price they have to pay. Equally, the motivation behind not wanting treatment may have to do with preserving the 'autonomy' of the person when ill, or, indeed, the existence of the ill person. Those who see value in the illness experience may want to ensure that they are able to continue to experience this.

Opting into treatment, however, may have more to do with preserving the autonomy of the well person. They, after all, are the only ones allowed to make the choice and they are choosing to limit the time they are ill. For most people this would be assumed to be the rational choice. Often they are also choosing the timing of the treatment as well as the type of treatment.

Since very few people opt out of all treatment but instead choose to limit the kinds or means of treatment, it is likely that some cost–benefit analysis, balancing treatment gains with side-effects and being ill, has been carried out at least informally by the patient.

The loss of autonomy of the person when ill does, however, require some consideration. If to have a mental illness means, at least part of the time, loss of autonomy, then a clear understanding of what is meant by 'autonomy' is needed. If patients are to have their liberty removed and receive possibly unwanted treatment because this autonomy has been lost, there is a need to establish why autonomy is so important and to whom it is important. If, in fact, autonomy is a central tenet not just of persons but of mental health there is a need to be clear about what is being attributed to the autonomy of the person that makes its loss so significant.

The importance of autonomy

Kant, in the *Groundwork of the Metaphysic of Morals* (1785, transl. Paton 1969), describes autonomy as 'the sole principle of ethics' and 'the ground of the dignity of human nature and of every rational nature' (p.97).

If Kant was right and not only human dignity, but also universal moral and ethical principles, stem from a regard for autonomy, then it is not difficult to understand why autonomy should be held in such high regard. Without it our moral system would collapse. In upholding autonomy as central to medical ethics, practitioners are preserving the dignity of the patient as a person by placing it in an unambiguous moral framework. By accepting the relationship of autonomy to morality they can know their decision has moral weight. The decision is beyond being merely pragmatic; it is right. It also means that in acting against it a moral decision is being taken, as well as a practical one. To be paternal, to decide to treat someone against their wishes, 'in their best interests', now becomes a moral act as well as a practical one.

It is this relationship between autonomy and morality which is vital to the issue of responsibility and the consequences for holding people with mental illness responsible or not for their actions. This may mean, in the most extreme cases, that they are found unfit to plead in a court of law for a criminal act they have committed. To a lesser degree they may be held not responsible for more minor acts of aggression against others or for acts of harm against themselves. If they are not morally responsible then we hold that it is inappropriate to punish them, but insist that they should be treated instead (see Chapter 8).

Autonomy is also a central tenet of utilitarianism, particularly when contrasted with paternalism, which Mill (1859, 1861) believed will (almost) never advance the interests of the individual. To develop morally and intellectually, to prefer 'the manner of existence which employs their higher faculties' (p.259) requires the person to have autonomy and self-determination and, further, requires society to promote these.

Utilitarianism is not without its problems in respect of autonomy, however. Matti Häyry's (1994) concerns for justice and rights 'are liable to put universal altruism into conflict with another set of values, namely freedom and autonomy' (p.82). To deal with some of these difficulties he proposed a theory of 'liberal utilitarianism'. This prioritises 'the necessary and basic needs for non-suffering, survival and autonomy' rather than 'particularised ethical intuitions or imperatives of intuitionist and deontological moralities'.

The nature of autonomy

Autonomy is the capacity for self-government and self-determination; the ability to choose for oneself. For an autonomous person their actions are truly their own. Self-determination requires an individual to have the capacity to formulate and carry out plans, desires and policies of their own devising. Self-government further requires the individual to take account of their own rules and values in making these choices. Thus desires and wishes may come into conflict with rules and values. Autonomy requires not only the mental and physical capacity to make choices and then carry them out, but also a social and political environment which cedes the importance and value of autonomy and allows it to flourish. Even within a society which values autonomy, choices and actions are both constrained and caused by external factors. If we add to this the external forces that shape physical, psychological and moral development then it would seem that no one is truly autonomous.

Feinberg (1986) described four closely related meanings of 'autonomy' when it is applied to the individual, namely the *capacity* to govern oneself as well as the *actual condition* from which springs an *ideal of character* and the *sovereign authority* to govern oneself within one's moral boundaries. It is 'capacity', however, which is the necessary underpinning for any of the other meanings. Feinberg noted that there are parallels with the term 'independent'. He further suggested that persons who are regarded as autonomous will also be regarded as having other virtues contingent on this. These are self-possession, self-identity or individuality, authenticity or self-selection, self-creation or self-determination, self-legislation, moral authenticity, moral independence, integrity or self-fidelity, self-control or self-discipline, self-reliance, initiative or self-generation and, lastly, responsibility for self.

Thus autonomy has limitations set on it, both by external and internal constraints, but also by the very nature of ideals of behaviour and attitude which it espouses. This self-reliance, as Feinberg noted, can become antisocial if it inhibits co-operation. There are usually social limits to self-creation. Performers such as Cher, Madonna or David Bowie may be able to reinvent themselves repeatedly, but such transformations may not be acceptable in other environments. Self-creation will almost certainly be deemed to have gone too far in those people who claim to be something or someone we cannot accept, whether this is an alien being or the reincarnation of Christ. The constraints on both the condition of self-governance and the 'ideal of character' will come largely from the desire for our own happiness, respect for others' autonomy and from the shared norms and beliefs of society at large.

Self-government is central to utilitarianism as described by Mill (1859, 1861). Within a liberal utilitarian philosophy Matti Häyry (1994), addressing 'need satisfaction', concluded that choices made by the autonomous individual are to be preferred to the choice made by the same individual who is not autonomous. This would seem to support advance directives.

The expression of autonomy, however, is a matter of degree depending, to a large extent, on external influences. What matters in this argument, however, are the consequences of assuming an individual does, or does not, have autonomy. If only autonomous beings are to be held responsible for their actions, then it is possible to escape blame and punishment if an individual can argue they were unduly influenced, i.e. were not acting autonomously. This will be discussed in Chapter 9.

If social and political external forces can confound autonomy so can other people in a more direct way. We need to distinguish here between those individuals who have the capacity to be autonomous, but whose ability to act on autonomous wishes is curtailed by, for example, slavery, and those who are heteronomous, whose will is controlled by others or who are otherwise under some external compulsion or constraint.

Thus physical illness may, in some cases, take away the ability to *act* autonomously but the person still has the *capacity* for autonomy, whereas in mental illness the capacity for autonomy is either questioned and denied or removed by the illness itself.

To deal with some of these problems there are conditions put on the individual before they can be deemed to be acting autonomously, or even to have the capacity to act autonomously. Chief among these is the need to act only under the influence of reason or rationality.

Who is autonomous?

The question 'who is autonomous?' can be clarified to mean who has the *capacity* to be autonomous rather than what conditions in society are necessary for a person to exercise self-government and self-determination. Heta Häyry (1991) suggested that, unlike self-determination, autonomy as *capacity* (or autarchy) is 'an all-or-nothing matter; either one has it or one does not have it' (p.58). This assumption will influence the answer.

Rational man is the clear answer to 'who is autonomous' provided by Kant (1785). Mill (1859), as described earlier, only applied his doctrine of self-determination to adults who do not require care from others. It may be supposed that Mill would include those who are mentally ill in the category of those who need to be 'taken care of by others'.

Feinberg (1986) acknowledged that the autarchic individual has the capacity to make foolish decisions as well as wise decisions. Among those unable to govern themselves, however, he cited 'lunatics' along with 'jellyfish, magnolia trees, rocks, new born infants...and irrevocably comatose former persons' (p.30). He went so far as to suggest that not only do these groups not have the capacity to govern themselves, they do not have the capacity to make decisions at all, even 'stupid' ones. 'Being stupid, no less than being wise, is the prerogative of the threshold-component' (p.30). Following this logic there is, however, as he points out, 'a kind of minimal compliment in being called "foolish"'(p.380).

There is arbitrariness about the inclusion of some of these groups into the company of the autonomous. Partly this is a result of autonomy being a maturational process. Mill relied on the law to fix an age for entry into adulthood. In Britain the right to vote is 18 years, the same age at which a person can order and drink alcohol in a public bar and watch all films. Since 16 years, however, this same individual has been able to join the army and learn to kill people and consent to sex and get married. Thus two more years of 'extra' maturity are required to vote for a government, an important act but one tempered by the vote of millions of others, than to make the, arguably more significant, individual choice of who and when to marry.

Considered developmentally it may be inevitable that autonomy is not 'all-or-nothing' as Heta Häyry (1991) claimed. In the adult, however, although it may be problematic to consider autonomy as a shifting state, this is likely to

reflect the reality. This is demonstrated in relation to capacity, for example, to consent to treatment.

Berofsky (1995) noted that the individual is not autonomous if they act 'out
of desires instilled in us by a hypnotist, demonic neurosurgeon or skilful manipulator' (p.209). If Berofsky was assuming that the person has not voluntarily
entered into these relationships, then there is a need to consider how far they can
over-ride autonomy. For example, there is widespread agreement that it is not
possible to hypnotise someone into carrying out behaviours they would not
engage in when not hypnotised, or do not want to do. The autonomous person
may, however, have chosen to enter hypnosis, or to have neurosurgery, because
they want the intended outcomes. This would be similar to what Szasz (1979)
described as psychiatry between consenting adults.

The definition of types of 'skilful manipulator' in this context may be important. Does skilled manipulation between health professionals and patients differ
to any great degree from the skilled manipulation found in other types of relationships? Indeed, a thorough analysis might demand an examination of the role
of 'manipulation' in most personal relationships. Is all persuasion in fact manipulation and a threat to autonomy? In a therapeutic relationship when does giving
information become manipulation?

To tell a patient that they will be committed to hospital involuntarily under a
section of the Mental Health Act unless they consent to be admitted voluntarily
may be viewed in a variety of ways. It can be seen as taking away any real choice
to voluntary admission. It can be seen as coercion in 'the patient's best interest' to
persuade them to enter voluntary admission and thus avoid the stigma of involuntary admission (although they lose the safeguards provided under the law). Or it
can be seen as a dispassionate assessment of the situation; the individual is going
to be admitted come what may, but they are being given a choice about how it
happens.

The question arises whether it is possible, or how and when it is possible, to
regain autonomy compromised by mental illness where there have to be interventions by another which may contravene the current wishes of the individual.
Advance directives may be seen as one way of maintaining autonomy by supplying capacitous decisions in readiness for a time of incapacity. Others may argue
that they compromise the autonomy of the ill person by tying them to previous
decisions – decisions to which they would not now, in their current state, wish to
adhere.

Autonomy and mental illness
People with mental illness, the 'lunatics' as they are called in some philosophy
texts, are usually dismissed from the realm of the autonomous with no

explanation. It is as though lacking autonomy has become, if not a symptom of madness, then at least a defining characteristic of it.

Problems arise, however, if there is no clear definition of what madness is, or who is to be called a 'lunatic'. In his discussion on autonomy and mental health Berofsky (1995) based his argument on those who are neurotic and, more specifically, those who have a phobia. Having accepted that a phobic person can be rational, that internal psychic conflict is not 'antithetical to autonomy', it is possible to choose to remain neurotic.

> ...the neurosis may be so satisfying, the pain of removal so great, and the dysfunctional condition so minor that the agent chooses to retain his neurosis, even after a rational review. He is deciding carefully and dispassionately, under complete information...He may see that it would be better to be different, but may not wish to pay the exorbitant price...But although his vision is influenced by his fears, it is not necessarily distorted. We cannot assume that this choice is not an autonomous one...There was a time when the choice to remain neurotic inevitably would have been looked on as just another sign of madness. Those times are thankfully behind us. One can choose rationally to be sick even on the assumption that the desire to be well is natural as universal (pp.207–8).

This exposition is clear but it does not help the understanding of autonomy in those individuals who choose to stay mad, where staying mad *is still* seen as a sign of madness. Berofsky demonstrated his confusion by avoiding being clear about what constitutes mental illness.

> I adopt the view that persons who are mentally ill can be autonomous so long as they meet the specific conditions: rationality, freedom, objectivity, independence and integrity. These conditions are, of course, not distinct from mental health. But it is not my task to consider the extent if any to which there can be autonomous people who are not mentally healthy. Our task is difficult enough without adding to it the project of defining mental illness (pp.224–5).

Thus mental health seems to be defined, at least in part, as meeting the condition of autonomy (and defining mental health is at least as difficult as defining mental illness).

If psychotic conditions are considered, then loss of autonomy is more an issue than in the 'neurotic' conditions, or what might be termed mental health problems. Psychosis is generally seen to interfere with autonomy, either as a symptom or a consequence of the illness. Some people who have a psychotic illness tell us unequivocally that they have lost their autonomy. Such individuals speak of 'having thoughts put in my head', 'having thoughts which are not mine' or 'being made to think something'. Other individuals, however, will claim to hear the voice of God, or an alien, or a dead parent or friend, who talks to them.

In the former case the individual is, if not claiming 'being taken over', at least recounting a series of events in their everyday lives which they experience as out-of-the-ordinary and not part of themselves. In the second scenario, however, even if the person comes to accept the experience as 'odd' (and they might not) it is, nevertheless, real to them, outside themselves and something to which they relate. In the first case the person will most likely agree that they are not autonomous in respect of the thoughts which are 'implanted', but may be autonomous in others. In the second case the individual may argue that they retain autonomy but that to exercise it is difficult because of the interference of the voices. It would be difficult for anyone to hold a conversation, maintain concentration or make decisions against a background of incessant, repeated monologue, often abusive and threatening. The Hearing Voices Network demonstrates this vividly in their training programmes for health professionals by having someone role play a voice hearer while another person is 'the voice' and keeps up the running commentary. In other cases people may report being 'compelled' to do what the voice was telling them, and thus experience this as loss of autonomy.

Throughout this discussion the concept of autonomy has not been challenged as a temporal issue; the focus has been on autonomy in the present. Advance directives, however, require a temporal view of autonomy: whether, when and why former preferences might have priority over current preferences. Developing the concept of precedent autonomy, Davis (2002) examines this in relation to living wills and people with dementia and in relation to subsequent consent (Davis 2004). Is it reasonable to base a medical decision on preferences a person is no longer able to affirm? He argues that in some cases it is, where these are highest-order values and the person's present condition, such as dementia, prevents them reflecting on their earlier preferences. Dresser (1982) had already made some consideration of this in relation to the Ulysses contract.

This might tie in with an approach to autonomy in the context of autonomy as authenticity rather than autonomy as sovereignty (or self-governance) where autonomy is protecting the self (Van Willigenburg and Delaere 2005). These ideas will be related to the concept of continuity of the person in Chapter 9.

CHAPTER 7

Personhood and Advance Directives in Mental Health

The legitimacy of an advance directive relies on the assumptions that the person who makes the advance directive and the person to whom it applies are the same and that the former has a right to decide what happens to the latter in some anticipatory sense. These assumptions raise a number of philosophical, ethical and practical questions.

A consideration of the philosophical requirements of being a person may sit uneasily with a clinical approach to 'personhood' and care giving. The latter focuses on a moral duty of care towards those in need of care (and who may or may not be a patient), whether this is between the cared for and care giver, or the approach of organisations to service provision. The emphasis is on the dignity, individuality and humanity of the person and has been expressed particularly in relation to people with dementia and learning disability but also applies to services for people with mental health problems. This will apply regardless of whether the individuals meet a philosopher's requirements for being a person.

The approach of Kitwood and colleagues (Kitwood and Benson 1995; Kitwood and Bredin 1992) to people with dementia has encompassed the current needs, wishes and preferences of the person. There may be good moral and practical reasons for prioritising the current wishes of the person with dementia over former, capacitous decisions in situations that affect their present comfort and quality of life, but not in others, such as disposal of wealth. The law remains clear that a person's last will and testament has to be made whilst capacitous and cannot be overturned by an incapable person.

It would not be possible, however, to apply this approach to dementia to all humans, irrespective of their capacity, without giving them the same status as persons. If capacitous and incapacitous individuals were to be treated equally as persons there would be no possibility for advance directives, for guardianship or any other safeguard for, or control over, people with incapacity. In this respect the concept of 'person' has more to do with issues of cognitive capacity and decision-making, of autonomy and responsibility. In some cases it might be more a question of language than underlying concept. Individuals judged incapable under the law are still, in most cases, referred to as 'persons', even though they may have been relieved of some of their rights to determine their own lives. Most people would probably still refer to an unconscious individual as a 'person', although this may be part of a series of states passing through coma to persistent vegetative state (PVS). The difference in this case is that the unconscious person is not trying to make a current decision for themselves, whereas the conscious but incapacitated person is.

To ignore some of the questions it is necessary to ask, because they seem insulting or politically incorrect, fails to safeguard individuals or ensure appropriate treatment or consideration. The rights of the person while ill (or incapable) must be reconciled with the rights of the person when well (or capacitous).

In relation to advance directives the question of what it means 'to be a person' goes beyond that of whether a person can make a capacitous decision. The question is whether the concept of 'person' differs in its sense when it refers to someone who is 'mad' rather than 'sane'.

A person who has made an advance directive, or a jurisdiction which allows advance directives, has, at least implicitly, answered some of these questions. The mad person is not the same as a sane person; the sane person's wishes take precedence over those of the mad person and the sane person is allowed to make decisions on behalf of the mad person. What, then, is it that justifies these assumptions? To answer this is to consider what it means to be a person.

Few philosophers discuss madness in their consideration of what it means to be a person. Some explicitly exclude this, usually on the grounds of irrationality, which is deemed central to the concept of person. Some are more extreme and go so far as to question the mad individual's status as a human being. Benn (1989) described those who do not achieve a minimal form of rationality (autarchy) as falling short 'in some degree as being a human being'. Schizophrenia is included, along with 'epistemic irrationality' and 'impulsion' as leading to autarchy. What this might mean to an individual so labelled is not discussed.

In examining the concept of person in relation to dementia Bourgeois (1995) never once suggested that the individual with dementia ceases to be human, although they may cease to be a person, or cease to be the person they once were. Bourgeois' approach and many of his ideas have been adapted here in relation to mental illness (or madness) although the philosophers themselves may not always consider this issue. Views of madness current at the time may have precluded them considering madness in this way. From the ancient Greeks until the end of the nineteenth century, with the emergence of the 'unconscious', madness was related to either punishment by God(s) or evil spirits or the work of the devil. It is unlikely, therefore, that a consideration of how mad individuals should be considered in relation to the concept of persons would be conducted within such a framework if it were used today.

The concept of 'person', as distinct from 'human being', stems from Roman philosophers building on and adapting ideas from the Ancient Greeks, notably Plato and Aristotle, who valued reason. It was not, however, until the seventeenth century that the concept of 'person' became a central problem for metaphysics as it became closely related to moral issues. Locke was particularly concerned with responsibility. Descartes' dualist approach separated the mind from the body, although somehow related to the body.

Writing about 100 years later Kant used the term 'person' in a similar way to Locke and it is from him that the current view of rationality as the fundamental characteristic of the person stems, although this has often lost its close link with the person as a moral being.

> Rational beings…are called persons because their nature already marks them out as ends in themselves – that is, as something which ought not to be used merely as means – and consequently imposes to that extent a limit on all arbitrary treatment of them (and is an object of reverence) (Kant 1785/1969, p.91).

The modern existential movement from the mid-nineteenth century was a revolt against the traditional metaphysical approach to man and his place in the universe and encompassed a number of different philosophers, including Kierkegaard, Jaspers, Heidegger and Sartre. Kierkegaard, the first of these, disputed the centrality of rationality to the nature of persons.

Some of these ideas will be visited in the following chapters. The focus of this chapter is on the continuity of persons through time since this is central to the concept of advance directives. Reason (or rationality) will be taken as an important defining characteristic in the concept of 'person'.

The concept of person and continuity of persons

Although for most of everyday waking life the concept of one person in one body, and the identification of the body as the person, are useful, there are times when this breaks down. Leaving aside the normal changes brought about through maturation and experience, there are the changes wrought by illness and trauma. There is not the space here to consider personhood and continuity in individuals with dementia or brain injury, nor changes brought about by long-term physical illness or as a consequence of addictive behaviours. The focus here is on people with a mental illness.

Families and friends make reference to the change in the individual: 'He's not the person he was', or 'She's changed out of all recognition', are common. People with mental illness, too, may see the changes and speak of 'not being myself when

I did that'. It does not necessarily follow that this applies only to states of disordered volition; it can apply to other aspects of the illness, including acting under the influence of delusions or hallucinations. Although many patients recognise that they have an illness, many do not and some may recognise it when they are 'well' but not when they are 'ill'. Psychosis is the only illness where refusal by an individual to accept they are ill can be taken as a confirming sign that they are. Clinically described as 'lack of insight' it clearly offers many opportunities for abuse for personal, social or political reasons.

'The person as they were before' – that is, before the illness took over – haunts therapy and management of people with severe mental illness. Some families perceive the change in their relatives as akin to bereavement, but with no body to mourn and a living stranger to get used to. Others see the change in their relative as temporary, with a new person replacing the old while the acute phase of the illness lasts. Although for some conditions, such as bipolar disorder, the personality usually remains intact, and the 'old' person does return, in other conditions, notably schizophrenia, repeated acute relapses take their toll and there may be a more or less gradual disintegration of the personality until only shadows of the 'previous person' are left. Both Kraeplin (1896/1919) and Bleuler (1911/1950) believed this to be an essential part of the illness. New drugs, the so-called atypical neuroleptics such as clozapine, have demonstrated that in some cases this is not true and much of the person can be restored (Degen and Nasper 1996).

If, as so many patients and relatives accept, there is a fundamental change in the person when ill, which possibly renders them a different person, how does this affect their writing an advance directive?

The common sense approach of one body–one person comes, as does so much of 'common sense', from Aristotle, to whom the concept of continuity was central. This view of the body as the living representation of the self and inseparable from it was developed by Wiggins (1967, 1980). He granted persons the status of a substance concept which applied to a being throughout their life. The person is only associated with the body during life; a dead body is not a person (although the body may still be valued and respected). The person is, however, more than just a living body, having, as it does, irreducible psychological properties such as reason and intellect, perception and emotion. The person remains the same person, even when intellect and reason are diminished. It would be possible, however, to argue that the person with no intellect and reason, but with lots of emotion and perception, is 'less' of a person, if reason is a priority in the definition of a person.

Williams (1973) also placed the person in their body, but did not identify the body with the person. There are, however, various types of person with different characteristics. Personhood is not a category whereby the satisfaction of certain degrees or levels of characteristics make an individual a person or not. Persons are sets of characteristics which may vary in degree over time and thus the person may change over time. Thus the mad person remains the same person, even though all may agree the characteristics which make up the person, or the ratio of them, have changed.

Locke took a different approach (1689/1948). He saw the continuity of the person as the same as the continuity of consciousness; one conscious state links the person to a previous conscious state. The substance in which the consciousness continues, however, may change over time. An important aspect of Locke's theory of consciousness which affects continuity of the person and personal responsibility is that consciousness has a sense of history and incorporates memory and knowledge of the past along with knowledge of the present and anticipation of the future. It is memory for the past that provides continuity for the person. A period of total amnesia in which the past is forgotten means that the individual is no longer the same person. If, however, the amnesia is selective and events prior to it can be remembered then there is the required continuity of consciousness.

This is relevant to the issue of conscience and responsibility. Being concerned with the resurrection of the body at the day of judgement, Locke suggested that persons have only done what they remember doing, and that persons should not be punished for actions they do not remember. Leaving aside all the very complex questions raised by psychologists relating to remembering, recalling and recognising, there are other problems with a theory which suggests that a person has only done that which they remember doing.

Parfit (1984) attempted a philosophical revision of Locke's philosophy. He argued that a person is a series of events, linked together by 'relation R'. He rejected the idea that a person's consciousness can split into two and suggested that if this happens the person is lost. R is the process by which experiences are chained together and it is not the person but the experiences and the process of R which are of most importance. Thus memories regain their status for personhood, and as long as there are overlaps, memory is continuous; it does not matter if some parts of the memory are lost. Madness does not affect memory in the way that dementia does and so the person could, arguably, remain the same.

Possibly the most interesting approach in relation to advance directives and mental illness is the theory of 'closest continuer' as proposed by Nozick (1981). The closest continuer does not simply resemble the original but is caused by the original. Thus the properties and characteristics of the original give rise to the properties and characteristics of the closest continuer. To define what is meant by 'closest' Nozick introduced a similarity metric made up of weighted dimensions. The metric is a means of bringing together causal and qualitative dimensions which make up the person. The dimensions can be any of the characteristics used to judge people and include both personality traits and physical properties. The dimensions are weighted with a character trait having more weight assigned to it than a physical characteristic such as brown hair. Identity is thus defined by the metric. Closeness depends on these weighted dimensions in relation to the metric. The metric, although it may vary between individuals in how they apply it, must be used by each individual consistently with all others. Thus the judgement of who is the 'closest continuer' is made in the same way, by each person, to all others.

There are, however, limitations to this theory. One of these is mono-relatedness. If the person continues there is not only a successor but a predecessor. For the closest continuer to be the person not only must they be the person's closest continuer but the original must be their closest predecessor. Although in the real world this may seem an unlikely problem there is a serious question of relation for those individuals who have episodic periods of mental illness. Is their closest predecessor the sane person who precedes the episode of mental illness or the ill person from the previous ill episode?

There are also metaphysical limits, which require that the class of persons should be as similar to each other and as dissimilar to non-persons as possible. This classificatory scheme can be widened or narrowed depending on how the concept of person is to be defined. Thus to include in the classification the ability to reason (or the capacity to develop this ability) narrows the concept and excludes those human beings who cannot reason, now or potentially.

Finally, there are social limits to how far we might incorporate others. Appropriating another's body parts as one's own is unacceptable, although we see this medically, and socially, sanctioned through transplantation and supported by informed consent.

Nozick allowed the individual to take part in determining who is their closest continuer. The person is created and recreated through the process of reflexive self-reference. This means that the person is able to recreate themselves as often as they like or society will tolerate.

For those who become mad two questions arise. Is madness a dimension and, if so, where does this fit in the metric? Second, does the recreation of the self as what others conceive of as mad come about through reflexive self-reference? The answer to the first question is open to debate; the answer to the second would seem to be 'no'. Madness brought about this way would make the adoption of madness conscious, whereas madness is generally thought of as being something which happens to the person. Whether it is the result of conscious volition or not will have an impact on the way the dimension of madness is weighted.

Nozick had four theories about identity over time. In the first identity follows the closest continuer, who is assessed by the weights given to different dimensions. Body, personality traits, cognitive abilities make up these dimensions. If reason is given over-riding weighting then this will make the reason-less being unlikely to be viewed as closest continuer. If, however, bodily characteristics are weighted more heavily, then the closest continuer will be that body. Since the individual themselves is involved in deciding who the closest continuer is, the metric involving reason might change. Thus the non-mad who fear madness may see themselves as ceasing to exist if they become mad, but once mad may accept their former self as their closest predecessor. Their metric might be revised later in line with their new information so that the changes wrought by madness are given less weight to allow the closest continuer to be the non-mad person.

The other theories apparently move into the realms of science fiction but they do allow for a more 'open' approach to the concept of who is 'the person'. The second theory proposes a solution to the problem of there being two contenders for the role of closest continuer. The solution provided is that the longest living is the closest continuer. Thus if the supposed closest continuer dies the next closest continuer takes over.

The third theory dispenses with the crossover and suggests that even though a less close continuer, the person continues in the longer lived contender. It is thus only in later stages of life that earlier stages are agreed as being part of the person or not. Lastly, there might be many contenders for the role of closest continuer as the person divides into many parts. The closest continuer is an amalgamation of some of these pretenders to closest continuer to form an actual continuer.

Although these theories may seem a little far-fetched they offer useful ways of considering a person who goes through stages of 'not being themself'. For example, is the mad individual the closest continuer until the non-mad person returns? Or, if it is known (expected) that the non-mad person will return, the mad individual is discounted because they are not the closest continuer, as in the third theory.

The fourth theory may assist in examining the problems inherent in ethical decisions in multiple personality, although therapy will be directed less towards maintaining the original than in integrating the personalities to create a new, 'whole' person.

In Nozick's terms the closest continuer might be the sane person, but this might be seen as denying the mad 'personhood' status as conceived in clinical practice terms. This means denying those individuals the right to make choices and decisions that meet that individual's or self's needs. There may be different ways forward here. One is to consider the nature of capacity, rationality and decision-making. Capacity is not an all-or-nothing quality and the person may lack capacity in some aspects of their life but not others. Another approach would be to consider the impact of the decision/choice on the person's current and future life. Thus decisions that will substantially impact on the person's future, such as treatment decisions, or financial or major relationship decisions, may be viewed more conservatively (i.e. to protect the future) than decisions which are seen as more trivial or transient. This would likely relate to capacity to make decisions as even people found legally lacking capacity may still be able to make reasonable and capable decisions over many everyday areas of life.

Thus medical decisions, or decisions about treatment, which for many are the main focus of advance directives, may be seen as being in a different category, for clinical staff who have to implement them, than other aspects of daily living.

Continuity of choices

A related, but different, approach would be to consider not the continuity of the person, but the choices which that person makes. In one of the few papers which considers the philosophical relationship between past, present and future choices (and which therefore deserves some detailed consideration) Savulescu and Dickenson (1998a, 1998b) argued strongly for the relevance of advance directives to people with a mental illness by bringing together two different philosophical arguments: one being to take a present-oriented approach and the other that preferences should be considered as dispositions.

Rejecting the framework of temporal neutrality, when preferences made at any time, for any time, are equal, and a present-only approach, which only considers present preferences, they opted for the present-oriented approach, particularly following Parfit (1984), which is weighted towards present preferences, but includes very close past and future preferences.

Thus, adopting the approach taken by Ryle (1963), they argued that preferences and desires are dispositions to act. That is, given certain circumstances a person has a disposition (a tendency) to act in a particular way (in relation to a particular set of circumstances). Crucially, the person does not have to be currently promoting that preference to maintain the disposition. Thus the disposition, or preference, to live might continue, although a person is presently engaged in risky behaviour. Whilst some might argue that the more rational preference should be respected (and Savulescu and Dickenson do not agree on this point) others might look for evidence for support of the preference by assuming gratitude on the part of the person in the very near future.

Furthermore, to be acted upon, the preferences stated must have existed at some point when the person was capable and fully informed. It does not follow that the person has to be capable now, or even to have the same dispositional preference. Interestingly Savulescu and Dickenson suggested that this means that the person need not have had capacity when the advance directive was made, so long as at some point they espoused the preference when capable. This is, however, unlikely to be persuasive for many clinicians or lawyers given current guidelines, and most jurisdictions require the person to be capable when making an advance directive.

This 'present-oriented dispositional analysis' gives rise, Savulescu and Dickenson (1998a) contended, to a number of implications for advance directives for people with a mental illness. The main contention is that 'advance directives are relevant insofar as they represent a person's present dispositional preference' (p.242). This suggests that where a non-capable position is supported by an advance directive, the advance directive gives emphasis to the present view which can then be treated as an autonomous view. It also suggests that although a person may currently have 'disordered and irrational preferences' as a result of psychosis, the views expressed in the advance directive may persist as present dispositions and therefore must be respected. This remains the case even if such preferences involve the person in 'greater than necessary risk, including the risk of self-harm or suicide'.

Thus to treat a person with an opt-in advance directive in the face of current refusal of treatment it would have to be assumed that the desire for treatment or to be 'well' was not only the current preference when the advance directive was made but is a *current* preference, albeit unexpressed and in the face of protestations to the contrary. Thus Savulescu argued for priority to be given to rational over irrational preferences, even where the latter are competent. The belief that the rational preference may be more important may come from experience of the person's past preferences as well as the knowledge of others in the same situation (for example, to adapt to changed circumstances).

Savulescu and Dickenson (1998a) also argued that the preferences of people with mental illness should be treated with the same respect as those with physical illness and to do otherwise is discriminatory. This includes refusing treatment. In relation to not being treated they argued against treating mental competence as having any special value. If, as they suggested, the reason for 'restoring a person to competence' is so they can decide on a course of action, then a 'settled competent dispositional preference' of refusal of treatment in an advance directive has already answered this decision and there is thus 'no reason to over-ride it'.

Although they make a distinction between 'irrational preferences which place the person at a greater risk of harm or death' (which they liken to people undertaking risky activities in everyday life) and advance directives which intend self-harm and death they do allow for 'suicidal advance directives' being respected 'if they are valid, clearly established, and applicable in the circumstances which result'. Indeed, they suggest that a suicidal advance directive is less of a problem than a present suicide attempt, as it allows time to address the concerns of those who object to allowing someone to die.

This leads to the somewhat perverse scenario which encourages someone to state that they want to be allowed to die with the express intention of talking them out of it. Although if someone does change their mind, it could be agreed that this was not an enduring dispositional preference, it does smack of deceit and manipulation in encouraging the advance directive in the first place.

Savulescu and Dickenson briefly considered whether the competent individual is the same as the non-competent using the notion of Parfit's 'psychological connectedness' rather than the notion of identity. Thus other future mental states are important in how they relate to current mental states. This allows for a future self to be so distant from the present self as to be another person. Since they have argued that advance directives should only be respected if the espoused preference endures in the present, it follows that in some cases, where the preference expressed is no longer important to the individual, it should not be respected. They went so far as to suggest: 'Perhaps we should treat future incompetent individuals as if they were individuals in their own right, according to what is in their interests at that time' (p.240).

Since, however, they illustrated this with the example of dementia it is not clear how far they intend this to apply to intermittent non-competent individuals as might be expected in mental illness.

Although their thesis is the relevance of advance directives in mental illness they draw on examples from physical illness and dementia, including persistent incompetence and terminal illness. This is both a strength and weakness as in doing so they apparently conclude that incompetence means different things in a transient and permanent state for how it reflects present dispositional preferences. Thus it might be reasonable to treat differently the advance directives of someone in a persistent vegetative state, with dementia or with intermittent mental illness. Although practically this might have some attractions, theoretically it causes problems for the concept of persons. This point was noted by both Dresser (1998) and Brock (1998) (both philosophers) in their commentaries on the papers.

Dresser (1998) also noted the problem of understanding the person's 'genuine preferences', and normative or objective restrictions on a person's advance directives remain the same under this as any other approach.

Brock (1998) further suggested that it is a 'serious theoretical misunderstanding' by Savulescu and Dickenson to treat advance directives only as evidence of earlier preference. Rather, he suggested, they are 'performance utterances' which depend on 'background social practices in order to create obligations and responsibilities'. Savulescu and Dickenson (1998b) dealt with this by suggesting that advance directives are 'not contracts in any relevant sense' as no other party is involved. Whilst it is true that no other party has to agree to a change (unless it is to confirm capacity) the advance directive does rely on another party to carry it out. Where the law gives weight to an advance directive, either to be considered (weaker case) or followed (stronger case) there is arguably some form of implicit contract. Some service users want this made much more explicit by giving advance directives full legal authority.

Somewhat worryingly Savulescu and Dickenson use as the example of someone independently changing their mind a man who in the past wanted to die if he became paraplegic but having become so, and being competent, changes his mind. Many people would want to honour this change of mind even if he were not competent.

Brock also had a number of practical concerns about implementing Savulescu and Dickenson's views. One was the suggestion that rational preferences were to be preferred when preferences conflict, and who was to decide this; another was the difficulty in knowing which dispositional preferences persist in the present if they are not being expressed; and lastly the difficulty of knowing what constitutes a true change of mind.

Burgess (1998) (a psychiatrist) also had concerns about managing a change of mind and described the present dispositional interpretation as 'a type of individualised substituted judgement' although Savulescu and Dickenson argued against it being that. Like them, however, she also rejected temporal neutrality, arguing that it is only the most recent preferences, which include the experience of mental illness, which reflect the person's whole understanding. With respect to observing advance directives which allow for suicide she was sceptical and suggested that this would be an 'unsafe position' and that clinicians who do so would put their 'career, as well as the patient's life, out on a limb'. For many, not just psychiatrists, this remains the sticking point with psychiatric advance directives.

Eastman (1998) (a barrister) focused on the relevance of the present dispositional position to the decisions made under the 1983 Mental Health Act in England and suggested that the "gated" ethical approach to the relationship between "autonomy" and "consequences" is probably not reflected in the "balance" approach taken by doctors and lawyers.

Many of the objections Savulescu and Dickenson (1998b) countered by reiterating their view are for a present-oriented approach and not a present-only approach. It is not always clear, however, when they talk about present preferences of 'the mentally ill' whether these are competent or incompetent preferences or, indeed, how competence is established. This is, in itself, surely a vital part of the process. They are themselves divided on the issue of the weighting to be given to rational preferences.

They do not deal with much of the reality of mental illness by equating choice with freedom, and likening a choice to refuse treatment to dying for 'the freedom of one's country'. They ask: 'Would it be better to experience mental illness and be free than to have one's mental illness under control but be institutionalised?' (Savulescu and Dickenson 1998b, p.263–6).

A practical objection to this is that if the person's mental illness *is* under control they are unlikely to be institutionalised (unless detained as a mentally disordered offender). It might be better to treat the argument as experiencing mental illness but living free from the side-effects of medication. Even here there are concerns. A competent choice might be made to stay ill rather than be treated. The problem arises, however, when the ill person is not able to make many of the important decisions in their life. By dismissing Mill's and Kant's views (Savulescu and Dickenson 1998a) that people should not be able to sell themselves into slavery, they seem to suggest that the person's own country of (incompetent) mental illness is preferable to the 'totalitarian country' of sanity (or treatment).

It is a romantic notion of mental illness that all people can live freely with mental illness and not come to harm, whether this is through neglect of their welfare by themselves or others, exploitation by others or active harm to themselves. Those that can will usually be left alone; it is those who cannot who usually come up against mental health legislation. To live safely and freely with their mental illness will require someone else to act for them in certain situations to prevent harm. Without this the free life might be one of squalor, homelessness, exploitation and possibly death. It is not clear that people who want to experience mental illness also want to experience this.

CHAPTER 8

Rationality, Decision-making and Advance Directives

Rationality or reason is at the core of many philosophical examinations of what it is to be a person, from Plato to Kant and later. Although there is normally a requirement for an advance directive to be made when the person is capable, there is not usually any (explicit) requirement for the decisions/directives to be rational. Where they are not, however, this might lead to the advance directive being challenged, based on the person's capacity, including being fully informed, when they made it.

One approach to rationality would simply be to ask, 'What criteria must be satisfied for a belief to be rational?' Another would be to ask, 'What is it that makes a rational person?'

Criteria for rationality

Nozick (1993), for example, set out six rules for rationality. The first of these is: 'Do not believe h if some alternative statement incompatible with h has a higher credibility value than h does' (p.85). Most mad beliefs, such as delusions, would fall at this first hurdle. The beliefs, for example, that an individual is being controlled by aliens, that the television can put a thought directly into a person's mind, or broadcast their thoughts, are trumped by scientific belief or knowledge.

There is, however, a tension between the theoretical and the practical. Nozick dealt with this by asserting the two principles: 'Do not believe any statement less credible than some incompatible alternative – the intellectual component – but then believe a statement only if the expected utility of doing so is greater than that of not believing it – the practical component' (pp.175–6).

This does not, however, deal with the issue of who is to decide what is credible. Rational belief is not, however, all or nothing. It has a 'cumulative force' whereby even very small differences in rationality will lead to a different belief or decision which will be compounded by the next very small difference, and so on.

Criteria for the rational person

Häyry (1991) related rationality more closely to the concept of personhood. She described conditions for the rational person as:

a) 'her beliefs form a coherent whole' (p.121);

b) 'her preferences form a coherent whole' (p.121);

c) 'her decisions and choices are consistent with these beliefs and preferences' (p.121);

d) 'her beliefs among themselves and her preferences among themselves are perfectly non-contradictory' (p.122);

e) 'she can give a clear account of how she reaches particular decisions and choices by collecting evidence and basing her conclusions on it' (p.122);

f) 'her decisions and choices are, to a reasonable degree at least, her own, i.e. they are not primarily the product of coercion, pressure or manipulation by others' (p.123);

g) 'she can act according to her own decisions and choices without explicit internal or external constraints' (p.124);

h) 'she can herself concretely accept the totality of her own decisions and choices, i.e. she can commit herself to them in her intended conduct' (p.124);

i) '(the most important of) her decisions and choices are designed, and can be expected, to further her own interests' (p.125);

j) 'typically makes (the most important of) her decisions and choices on the grounds of what (she thinks) is moral' (p.126);

k) 'she is willing to live according to the rules of a given just society' (p.126);

l) 'she has good reason to believe that the majority of her beliefs are essentially correct' (p.126).

These conditions form 11 types of rationality, namely:

1. minimally rational or autarchic = a, b, c;

2. fully consistent = a, b, c, d;

3. explicitly rational = a, b, c, e;

4. autonomous = a, b, c, f;

5. free in a technical sense = a, b, c, g;

6. free in a moral sense = a, b, c, d, g, i;

7. possesses personal integrity = a, b, c, d, h;

8. prudential in the narrow sense = a, b, c, d, i;

9. moral = a, b, c, d, j;

10. a concrete historical person = a, b, c, d, k;

11. ideal decision-maker = a, b, c, d, l.

These conditions for types of rationality can be examined from the perspective of madness to see explicitly what it is that the mad lack and the sane possess. If it is accepted that no one completely fulfils the criteria all the time, even to being minimally rational, then it must also be accepted that minimal irrationality is part of the human condition. The question is thus turned around – not how irrational do you have to be to be considered mad, but how rational do you have to be to be considered sane?

Within these conditions the mad may be both autarchic and non-autarchic. Most of the mad individual's beliefs and preferences will be no different from the sane. 'Mad' beliefs frequently form only part of the individual's belief system, although they may be central and influence other aspects of the system. Conversely, in some people with paranoid delusions the false belief is encapsulated and does not interfere with other aspects of the individual's life, thus enabling them to maintain a degree of 'normality' in their life. In either case the problem may be less with the ability of the person to think rationally within their frame of reference than it is with the beliefs or premises on which the person is basing their decisions, which may not accord with the majority belief.

These conditions and types of rationality are helpful in separating the way in which a person thinks, and the structures of their beliefs and decision-making, from the content of those beliefs. To consider how these criteria might be examined in relation to treatment decisions, either in the present or in advance directives, it is worth considering an example of three men.

James has schizophrenia, accepts the diagnosis and acknowledges there are periods when he is ill, behaves in a way he normally would not and needs to be kept safe.

Jim also has schizophrenia but does not agree that he is ill. What others identify as episodes of illness he sees as periods when other people will not leave him alone to live his life as he wishes. He does, however, acknowledge that he has some problems 'fitting in'.

Malcolm has cancer. He has had surgery and chemotherapy. He has secondaries and there is no further curative treatment.

All three men have the same beliefs:

1. it is better to live than to die

    but

2. quality of life is more important than mere existence.

Also

3. it is better to be well than ill

    but

4. the consequences of treatment can be worse than living with an illness.

All three men want to refuse treatment, now and in the future: James and Malcolm for similar reasons. The side-effects of treatment are unacceptable. Malcolm would rather accept palliative care and die sooner, but enjoy a better quality of life with his family, than undergo further debilitating treatment for a longer period of life but much of it spent with increased suffering. James prefers to 'feel himself' when well, and would rather have a period of being kept safe in hospital when ill than to have the debilitating and disabling side-effects of medication which he previously experienced.

Jim is refusing treatment on the grounds that he is not ill and therefore there is nothing to treat. Like James he also found the side-effects of medication debilitating.

How far do these men meet the criteria for a rational person? All three may well meet the first five of Häyry's conditions. The first hint of difference may come with condition (f), that decisions and choices are predominantly that of the person. Although Häyry only considers pressure from others, the external impact of the illness may be a pressure on Jim. This requires an agreement that lack of insight is a symptom of schizophrenia. Thus all three reach the third type of rationality, but only James and Malcolm are autonomous (4). Although all men may experience external constraints in the form of pressure from family, friends and health care staff to accept treatment they can still choose to ignore it. It is here that the major differences between the men start to show. Both James and Jim may find treatment thrust upon them through mental health legislation. Malcolm cannot be forced to accept treatment. Depending on the legal criteria even James and Jim may find themselves treated differently. Under Scottish law, for example, James may be found to have the ability to make medical decisions, but Jim may not. Only Jim could then be compulsorily treated.

All three, however, meet the next condition (h). It is condition (1), acting to further one's own best interests, which may give rise to more problems. All three are acting in what they believe to be their best interest as laid out in the beliefs above. The key issue here is who is to decide what is in a person's best interest. The sane may believe that being mad is, by definition, not in a person's best interest. This would be one reason for forcing treatment on them. This may not be echoed by the mad. Even if being mad is not optimal, it may be viewed as less bad (for some of the time) than the impact of treatment, which may persist most of the time. The importance of quality of life rather than simply length of life has been accepted in many ways for the elderly, those with a terminal condition or major disability. Quality of life set against periods of madness is something people seem unwilling to apply in psychiatric conditions.

All three may believe they are making a moral choice in some way: Malcolm and James in choosing to retain their sense of self rather than be diminished by treatment and Jim in refusing what he believes to be unnecessary treatment. A further issue might arise if either of them were a risk to others when ill, but this will be pursued in Chapter 9.

The final two conditions and the types they embrace put rationality within a communitarian framework. In being a concrete historical person or citizen the individual is willing to live by the rules of a given just society. It is important to remember that the mad individual will conform to many, if not most, of the rules of a just society. It is the beliefs which conflict with either of these rules or, more accurately in many instances, the known facts as society perceives them (particularly regarding science and religion) that are defined as irrational, or mad. If these are kept private, or are encapsulated, then the individual may still live in society, undetected. The more these beliefs cause the person to act in ways which bring them into conflict with society's rules or conventions, the 'madder' they will be perceived.

James and Jim may not be willing to accept rules which allow them to be treated against their will. They may want to argue that such rules, or laws, are, in fact, antithetical to a just society.

For the last condition and type, decision-making is used in a technical sense to mean that the person believes the majority of their beliefs to be correct. In the West science tends to be the final arbitrator for many beliefs and choices and the experimental method the technique of choice for determining truth or fact. Where science does not hold the ultimate truth, for example, in matters of religion and faith, the majority or consensus view, based on long tradition, holds sway. It is this consensus which allows judgements of attitudes, beliefs, morals and actions to be judged correct, more-or-less correct or, in lay terms, 'mad'.

Although all three men may believe their beliefs to be correct it is Malcolm who will probably have the strongest agreement with others. James may receive some sympathy for his position, but the prevailing view is likely to be that he would be better off being treated. It is Jim, however, who will fall foul of the consensus view.

Malcolm's rationality is confirmed through all conditions and types of rationality. James is much more rational than not. He only falls at the 'concrete historical person' because of problems of living with the rules of a just society. Even Jim turns out to be at least as rational as he is not, and even here the problem is with what he believes, not how he thinks about it.

Imprudence

Häyry (1991) concluded her definitions of rationality by describing its opposite: 'imprudential in the widest sense'. This applies if the person 'lacks autarchy, autonomy, personal integrity, prudence in the narrow sense, morality, historical rationality, or one of the qualities of the ideal decision-maker' (p.127).

Although Häyry accepted that to be fully consistent and rational is unlikely to be achieved by most individuals, she nevertheless suggested that 'if any one of the genuinely essential and intrinsic characteristics of rationality' are missing the individual can be charged with 'imprudence'.

Is this all madness turns out to be, imprudence? At the very least a clinical definition of madness would suggest not, and even cultural definitions are unlikely to settle simply for this. Nor is the law. The Mental Health (Care and Treatment) (Scotland) Act 2003 excludes 'acting as no prudential person would act' from the definition of mental disorder (Section 325).

Where, however, decisions about treatment and care (including those made in an advance directive or by proxy decision-makers) are expected to be based on a 'best interest' judgement then imprudence is likely to be cited as irrational when decisions do not conform to best interest.

Individual and community rationality

Following these rules for rationality, however, may be seen by some as little more than following rules for reasoning or logical thinking or behaviour and there is no real argument that even mad people cannot argue rationally or logically within their particular 'mad' framework. Locke (1689/1948) argued this in *An Essay Concerning Human Understanding* (Book II, Chapter XI). He contrasted 'idiots' who are 'deprived of reason' with 'madmen' who

> ...seem to suffer by the other extreme. For they do not appear to me to have lost the faculty of reasoning, but having joined together some ideas very wrongly, they mistake them for truths; and they err as men do that argue right from wrong principles. For, by the violence of their imaginations, having taken their fancies for realities, they make right deductions from them...Hence it comes to pass that a man who is very sober, and of a right understanding in all other things, may in one particular be as frantic as any in Bedlam...In short, herein seems to lie the

difference between idiots and madmen: that madmen put wrong ideas together, and so make wrong propositions, but argue and reason right from them; but idiots make very few or no propositions, and reason scarce at all (p.62).

Discussing further distinctions between 'right' and 'wrong' ideas Locke concluded that we all observe 'something that seems odd...in the opinions, reasonings, and actions of other men' (p.196). Although accepting that this 'sort of unreasonableness' can be attributed to education and prejudice, Locke goes further, calling it both a disease and madness.

> I shall be pardoned for calling it by so harsh a name as madness, when it is considered that opposition to reason deserves that name, and is really madness; and there is scarce a man so free from it that he should always, on all occasions, argue or do as in some cases he constantly does, would not be thought fitter for Bedlam than civil conversation. I do not here mean when he is under the power of unruly passion, but in the steady calm course of his life (p.197).

This was not a fashionable view in its day and McCrone (1993) suggested that Locke was describing madness as 'an altered state of consciousness' (p.212). This would find support today from a variety of sources, but not necessarily using the same line of reasoning.

Locke's description of madness as 'a weakness to which all men are so liable ...a taint which so universally infects mankind' (p.197) does not accord with clinical definition which describes a dichotomy between psychotic illness and non-psychotic. It might, however, be more in touch with the current view of mental illness as part of a continuum, rather than as a dichotomy. In either case, however, psychosis is limited to a minority of individuals. It does, however, realistically describe the prevalence of 'everyday irrationality' or 'everyday madness'. Locke clearly situated madness in the realm of thought and the association of ideas rather than emotions. For Locke the loss of reasoning was not the inability to be internally consistent, but that the mad have 'wrong ideas' which lead them to 'wrong propositions'.

Nozick (1993) suggested rationality can correct biases in information and questioned how wide such scope for correction is. He asked whether individuals are limited to 'the range of options about belief and action that our society presents to us' or whether it is possible to go beyond this and consider all options, all reasons for and against and in so doing correct 'for any biases we can detect due to the social transmission of information and the social weighting and evaluation of reasons' (p.128). Nozick opted for the latter option, although conceding that if options are equally matched, social values and determinates can be allowed to determine the outcome.

Where does this leave the mad? They may believe that they are rationally considering evidence and options from first principles, free of social bias and by reaching their own conclusions are exerting not only their rationality but their autonomy of decision-making. The rest of society may merely consider them wrong or may consider them mad. Copernicus and Galileo brought down the wrath of the Catholic Church by proposing a helio-centred universe rather than a geo-centred universe. They might have been considered both heretical and mad, but they were right. The fact that at the end of the twentieth century one-third of British and one-half of American adults did not know the earth revolves around the sun (reported in Brennan 1992) does not alter the evidence in any way or make the belief any the less wrong. It might, however, raise a question as to what counts as evidence.

Irrationality

Irrationality of the everyday type is generally distinguished from madness. Despite the colloquial use of the term, exclamations of 'I must have been mad' to explain a choice or behaviour later regretted or marvelled at do not normally indicate the person believes they were ill. Rather, they may believe the behaviour or choice was uncharacteristic or imprudent or irrational based on their usual beliefs. In everyday irrationality the cause may be incompetence and misinterpretation of conscious or unconscious wishes (Pears 1986). These may lead to self-deception or lack of self-control. A discussion of 'common-or-garden irrationality' (Sutherland 1992) or 'everyday irrationality' (Gardner 1993; Pears 1986) is outwith the scope of this book. It may, however, be useful when considering the types of decisions which people make in advance directives.

The important distinction which Pears (1986) made is that misperception of things in the external world is not the same as irrationality. Pears argued for two different cases of the influence of wishes. In the first the wish acts to bias or distort the process of belief-formation from the rational to the irrational. This may approximate to a condition of self-deception. In the second the bias or distortion is between the process of rational deliberation and action, which may approximate to a condition of lack of self-control. For philosophers the more important question may be how can people knowingly act against their own better judgement or best interests or whether self-deception is possible. Psychologists, on the other hand, usually assume that everyday experience shows us people doing this all the time and are thus more interested in finding out why they do this and how they can (be helped to) change. The philosophical approach involves identifying the true agent with their reason, so to act irrationally is to act against one's true self.

The paradox of irrationality requires the belief, at the same time, of two logically incompatible propositions or acting against one's beliefs. One way of explaining the irrationality would be to have a person consist of two sub-systems.

The main system would control both daily life *and* the irrational belief and all the information which makes it irrational. A sub-system would include the cautionary belief, which would be that, with the information the person had, it was irrational to form the belief they favoured. Had the cautionary belief been in the main system, then the irrational belief would not have been formed. Since, however, it belongs to the sub-system, it could not fulfil its cautionary role.

Pears (1986) suggested that this model is not required for irrationality 'at the bottom end of the scale, where it may be enough to observe that it is a common human failing to form beliefs unsupported by the evidence' (p.68). It is only at the extreme that we may need to suggest that a single person can have two independent systems operating at the same time.

In these explanations of irrational action the cause, or fault, lies in the deliberations of the agent. The original fault was an intellectual fault, albeit a motivated intellectual fault. The same wish that produced the intellectual fault produced the irrational action. An intellectual fault lying outside an agent's reasoning would be compulsion.

Pears related the backward connection between a non-compulsive intentional action and the agent's value judgement to the psychological theory of attribution, which suggests that 'rationalisation' is used to explain both the actions of the self and others. The connection is thus from doing to valuing. Even the forward connection from valuing to doing does not get rid of the problem of some forms of motivated irrationality.

In an apologia for his book Pears (1986) suggested that a common excuse 'for an unrelieved discussion of deviations and abnormalities' is that 'the investigation of the abnormal throws light on the normal' (p.257). This, however,

> ...is not true of the kind of irrationality that has been examined here. When a wish distorts normal processes of thought or the normal transition from thought to action, it works like an expert in demolition. The methods used may be interesting but they reveal very little about the structure that buckles and collapses under the attack. There is here a marked contrast with the unmotivated perversions of reason. A thorough study of those faults would lead in many cases to an analysis of logical fallacies sufficiently detailed to throw some light on valid reasoning (p.257).

Nowhere in his book did Pears mention madness, presumably because the irrationality of madness is unmotivated and does not stem from self-deception or incompetence or lack of self-control (in relation to actions and beliefs). Gardner (1993) also excluded from his discussion of irrationality that which arises from madness, along with error, incompetence and problems of self-knowledge or resolving value conflicts.

The psychologist Sutherland (1992) likewise ignored 'the effects of brain injuries or severe mental illness on rationality' (p.10) in his book *Irrationality*. Although stating that 'schizophrenia has devastating effects on rationality' he pointed out that 'psychologists know very much less about irrational behaviour caused by mental illness or by brain damage then they do about common or garden irrationality to which every one of us is prone' (p.11). What then, is the irrationality of madness?

The irrationality of madness

The irrationality of madness has little, if anything, to do with wishes and desires which lead to irrational beliefs and acts, but is a belief held as a fact which others believe to be irrational or untrue as a matter of fact. It is both involuntary and unmotivated. It must be distinguished from involuntary irrationality in the systems described above, which still hinge on a belief which is subjected to motivation (Sturdee 1995).

Generally speaking, the irrational beliefs of the mad have been assumed to be meaningless and unmotivated and would seem to fall into the category which Pears (1986) would deem merely incorrect. Such beliefs have also been assumed to be not amenable to argument, persuasion or therapy. The latter assumption may be open to question and this may force a reconsideration of the former assumption.

The advances in cognitive therapy with people with schizophrenia show some evidence that irrational beliefs are capable of modification through a process of rational challenge and accepting that the beliefs may have some meaning (Kingdon and Turkington 1994, 2004). There is also evidence from people who have 'returned from madness' following treatment with the new atypical antipsychotics (such as clozapine) that repressed memories of abuse and other traumas may have been incorporated in some way into the illness process (Degen and Nasper 1996). In other cases the abuse has not been repressed but has never been acknowledged to mental health professionals because it has never been asked about. The irrational perceptual experience which is hearing voices has been described by some of those in the Hearing Voices Network (www.hearing-voices.org) as both having meaning when it is deconstructed or interpreted and also amenable, in some cases to management, by the individual (Romme and Escher 2000; Thomas 1997). All these approaches challenge the belief that the defect of irrationality in madness is immutable. If it is true that 'mad irrationality' is capable of change then very difficult questions arise concerning the responsibility of the individual for acts which stem from these irrational beliefs and for which the individual has chosen not to accept treatment.

Returning to Locke (1689/1948) may be helpful, and making a distinction between reason, which is method or process, and rationality, which is about content and choice. Reason is thus how evidence is used to support choice; rationality is about what counts as evidence or influences the choice or goal. The three men described in this chapter, James, Jim and Malcolm, all want a 'rational' goal – quality of life. All employ a reasoned process to reach their decision to pursue a course of action to reach that goal. The problem arises with Jim because, for most people, the evidence (that he is not ill) is unacceptable and not rational. For James, the problem is that for some, possibly many, the choice to be ill rather than take psychotropic medication is irrational. This contrasts with Malcolm, where a similar action is seen as rational. This may be because the negative consequences are better known than for psychotropic medication, or because he is only postponing death by a short while. James, on the other hand, may avoid periods of sickness. The evidence for this will be interpreted differently by different groups.

This still does not give a clear method as to how to distinguish all beliefs which are to be deemed mad. Sometimes the intuitive belief of the majority is at odds with the evidence and rational process and the latter is simply abandoned. One example of this was the celebration of the millennium. Technically, it was argued, the new millennium started on 1 January 2001 (only then having completed 2000 years). For most people, however, the change from 1999 to 2000 looked 'right' and thus the new millennium started one year early, indicating that society does not always champion the rational over the emotional or intuitive. This contrasts with personal birthdays, which are celebrated at the end of the completed year, suggesting that contradictory reasoning is acceptable to most people depending on the circumstances.

There is also that uncomfortable group of beliefs which the majority do not accept, largely on the grounds of lack of, or contradiction to, current scientific evidence, yet believing in them does not lead the person to the label mad (but possibly eccentric). Leaving aside mainstream religious belief (which for much of history and in many parts of the world is the belief of the majority) we can cite beliefs ranging from UFOs and alien abduction to out-of-body experiences or the belief that Elvis Presley is alive, well and living in happy obscurity. It is difficult to know with some beliefs, such as conspiracy theories, which came first, the 'irrational' view of the evidence or the irrational theory of conspiracy which prompted the search for the evidence.

Although many proponents of such theories may be dismissed, colloquially, as 'mad', it is unlikely that many have fallen victim to mental health laws for that alone. Indeed, it could be argued that if someone were targeted, particularly by government agencies, for promoting a conspiracy theory, then that, in itself, would lend weight to the conspiracy theory and thus to it being a rational belief rather than irrational. (This might, however, be more indicative of the author's own powers of paranoid reasoning than real evidence.)

What makes the difference between someone who believes Elvis is still alive and the other types of delusional belief is the understanding of the origins of the belief. Where the belief, or choices, or decisions are interpreted by others as stemming from illness they will be deemed irrational and can be dismissed. Why and how lack of insight is different from denial, which occurs in many illnesses (or, indeed, the denial of Elvis' demise) is beyond this analysis. It is, however, central to how an advance directive will be received. A well reasoned directive would still fall, deemed as not competent, if the underlying premises were seen as irrational.

CHAPTER 9

Responsibility
and Its Consequences

Making an advance directive is as much about taking responsibility as it is about exerting autonomy. Where there is a choice there is also responsibility for that choice. There are two interconnected aspects to this responsibility. The first is the responsibility for treatment for the management of the illness and the consequences of that decision. The second aspect is the well person taking responsibility for the ill person and their actions.

Opting into treatment may have as much to do with concern over what the person does when ill, and wanting to prevent this, as it does with the actual treatment choices themselves. The well person may only be seeking to prevent harmful consequences (to themselves or others) because of the negative impact to themselves or they may believe they are responsible for the harm if they have not done all they can to prevent it.

Those who opt out, or limit, treatment because they do not like the side-effects of medication, for example, may be more concerned about the impact on themselves than the consequences for others. There are three separate issues here. The first is any harm visited on themselves by not taking treatment, and it might be agreed that the capacitous person has the right to make this choice. The second is the impact of continued ill health on service provision and the cost of this as borne by society. The question of how far people can be held responsible for lifestyle choices (and it could be argued that this is a lifestyle choice) has been raised in relation to the NHS in Britain in several fora recently (Halpern and Barnes 2004; Nuffield Council on Bioethics 2006). The third is the harm to others. If harm occurs to another person because of the well person's choice not to be treated, then how far is the well person responsible for their actions when ill?

Although a consideration of responsibility to advance directives must be taken against this backdrop, this is not the usual approach to responsibility and mental illness. The focus is more commonly on moral responsibility, particularly in relation to criminal acts. Elsewhere philosophers have 'written off' those with a mental illness as not responsible, with no real consideration of their capabilities or capacities. For example:

> Mere animals, who lack reason, are not responsible for their actions; nor are people who are mentally 'sick' and not in control of themselves. In such cases it would be absurd to try to hold them accountable. We could not properly feel gratitude or resentment toward them, for they are not responsible for any good or ill they cause. Moreover, we cannot expect them to understand why we treat them as we do, any more than they understand why they behave as they do. So we have no choice but to deal with them by manipulating them, rather than by addressing them as autonomous individuals. When we spank a dog who has urinated on the rug, for example, we may do so in an attempt to prevent him from doing it again – but we are merely trying to 'train' him. We could not reason with him even if we wanted to. The same goes for mentally 'sick' humans (Rachels 1986, p.136).

There is no attempt to suggest that the person is not responsible only some of the time, or only in some circumstances. The 'mentally sick' seem to be treated as an all-or-nothing category. This is not helped by the concept of mental illness, or even madness, not being defined, or drawn more widely than it would be clinically.

Wallace (1994) took an apparently similar view in dismissing the insane as being morally responsible, along with other groups such as children and, possibly, certain animals, and later includes conditions such as 'addiction, posthypnotic suggestion, behaviour control, psychopathy, and the effects of extreme stress, deprivation or torture' (p.166). Not everyone would agree with this, and Wallace pointed out that it may later be found that not all these categories are legitimately to be excluded. Mental illness, for example, may or may not exist in a particular way, but he took his argument from the position that if it does exist, and it is taken as a legitimate exemption from moral responsibility, then it is because its nature is defined in a way which makes it legitimate. In this case, he described the nature of mental illness as interfering with the power of reflective self-control.

Smiley (1992) argued that for the person 'so compelled by mental demons that she does not know who she is or what she is doing, we are all likely to excuse her from blame on the grounds that her will was not free' (p.228).

This leaves many actions by people with a mental illness in an ambiguous position. How is the behaviour of John Morrison, a man with a major mental illness, to be characterised when he dragged a drowning woman from Newhaven Harbour (Scotland), resuscitated her and stopped a passing car to telephone for assistance? Lothian and Borders Police certainly held him responsible, presenting him with a meritorious award for bravery (National Schizophrenia Fellowship (Scotland) 1997).

The notion of responsibility or its absence in mental illness is central to criminal law but implied rather than overt in civil law. Indeed, in many books dealing with aspects of civil mental health law responsibility does not even appear in the index (e.g. Appelbaum 1994; Eastman and Peay 1999; Fennell 1996; Winick 1997). Although an understanding of what constitutes being responsible for a criminal act is not central to making an advance directive it may offer some insights into the relationship between responsibility and madness.

Responsibility and the insanity defence

For a person to be found guilty of a crime under British law (and those systems based on it) they have to fulfil two conditions. First, they have to have committed a criminal act (the *actus reus* or bad deed) and, second, they have to have a criminal mind (*mens rea* or evil mind). The aim of the insanity defence is to demonstrate that the individual does not have *mens rea*; they are not bad but mad. It is not, however, a defence in the sense that self-defence can lead to acquittal. Since the Criminal Lunatics Act of 1800 in England, acquittal on the grounds of insanity does not lead to release (as it would with self-defence) but to commitment to a non-penal establishment. The insanity defence means detention and the removal of liberty for an indefinite length of time and, in many cases, longer than if the person had been sane and received a custodial sentence.

The various legal tests of insanity, such as the M'Naghten rules, are based on a number of explanations for behaviour which exclude responsibility. This stems from Aristotle's *Nicomachean Ethics* which grounded moral responsibility in voluntariness or intentional action (Elliott 1996). The two types of excuse which come from this are ignorance and compulsion. To these Reznek (1997) wanted to add a third category, 'change in moral character', the individual being 'transformed from a good character into an evil one' (p.309), the change being a result of the mental illness. He suggested that many juries already use this as a criterion in judging insanity.

This latter category raises the question whether mental illness can cause a change of character irrespective of criminal actions. This might or might not carry overtones of blame or moral responsibility or other sorts of responsibility for decisions and actions and play a part in the justification for mental health laws and treatment without consent.

Sanity and responsibility

One approach is that of Wolf (1987) who considered sanity and responsibility from the 'deep-self view' of responsibility. She argued that for some people 'the connection between the agents' deep-selves and their wills is dramatically severed' (p.50) when they are governed by independent, external forces, including hypnosis and brainwashing, or by conditions such as kleptomania. Although Wolf argued that there are multi-levels of deep-self and deep desires which convey freedom, she suggested that in order to be responsible the deep-self has to be sane, and called this the sane deep-self view in contrast to the plain deep-self view. Those who have insane deep-selves can try to take responsibility but it is, properly, only a characteristic of sane selves.

The problem with this argument as presented by Wolf is her, admittedly acknowledged, 'specialised' definition of sanity. This stems from use of the M'Naghten Rules as the criteria for sanity. This is a legal, not clinical, judgement and there is room for confusion between a legal concept of insanity and a medical concept of mental illness. Wolf compounded the confusion by the notion of the 'desire to be sane', which suggests some choice. She moved from the M'Naghten Rule of the person knowing what they are doing to interpreting this as a chain of beliefs from 'a desire to know what one is doing', to 'a desire to live in the real world', to 'a desire to be controlled (to have in this case one's beliefs controlled) by perceptions and sound reasoning that produce an accurate conception of the world, rather than by blind or distorted forms of response' (p.55).

The second part of the M'Naghten Rules, the understanding of right and wrong, Wolf interpreted as 'one's hope that one's *values* be controlled by processes that afford an accurate conception of the world' (p.55). Sanity, then, is 'the minimally sufficient ability cognitively and normatively to recognise and appreciate the world for what it is' (p.56), although she accepted that for some purposes 'this would be an implausibly broad construction of the term' (p.56). Although this definition may equate with a lay view of madness and, in some instances, with mental illness, it is her insistence that sanity 'involves the ability to know the difference between right and wrong' (p.56) that causes problems. This is a moral assessment not usually evident in clinical assessment or practice.

This view led Wolf to conclude that 'victims of deprived childhoods as well as victims of misguided societies may not be responsible for their actions' (p.57). In the latter she included 'the slaveowners of the 1850s, the Nazis of the 1930s, and many male chauvinists of our fathers' generation' (pp.56–57). Such people are, 'at the deepest level unable cognitively and normatively to recognise and appreciate the world for what it is. In our sense their deepest selves are not fully sane' (p.57). It is not that the views or values of such people are mistaken that is the issue, but that the person cannot avoid having those views/values.

The deep-self view holds that not only does the deep-self govern the superficial self, it also gives the individual the capacity to question what they want to be and what they want to change. Individuals are thus, Wolf asserted, morally, if not metaphysically, responsible for themselves since they could, if they wanted, change their characters and actions in an appreciation of what is right and wrong. Since the insane are unable to evaluate themselves 'reasonably and accurately' they do not have one of the required abilities for responsibility.

Wolf dealt with two problems with the sane deep-self view. First, the problem of how the individual can know that they are saner than the non-responsible, and second, whether this approach implies that everyone who acts wrongly or has false beliefs is not responsible. The first she answers by suggesting that the only thing which justifies it is agreement between individuals and success in negotiating the world and meeting their needs. That sanity is thus a normative concept she sees as a 'strength' in that 'severely deviant behaviour, such as that of a serial murderer or a sadistic dictator, does constitute evidence of a psychological defect in the agent. The suggestion that the most horrendous, stomach-turning crimes could be committed only by an insane person...must be regarded as a serious possibility...'(p.61). She does not consider evil as a possible reason for such behaviour, which may at least be a possibility (Morton 2004).

It is not only crimes, however, that can be discounted in this way, but '*any* wrong action or false belief' can be used as evidence that the individual does not have 'the ability cognitively and normatively to understand the world for what it is' (p.61). Although Wolf accepted that lack of this ability may be an explanation, there may be others, and other aspects of the person's life will aid deciding which explanation is most appropriate.

Wolf is not alone in reaching a point which seems to excuse people at the extremes of behaviour. Watson (1987), for example, in considering whether to be held morally responsible one has to be part of the moral community, concludes that those not being part of the community could lead to 'the paradox...that extreme evil disqualifies one from blame' (p.268).

Feinberg (1970), in considering mental illness and sickness, looked at the 'proper functioning' of the body and related this to conscience:

> Surely, there is one obvious sense in which no person can function 'properly' if he has no conscience. And one might argue that any person who commits batteries, rages, and murders is not in 'good working order' and that certain moral norms, therefore, must be included among the criteria of proper functioning (pp.256–7).

Wolf (1987) did not really question whether those she labels not responsible, such as Nazis, slaveowners and even male chauvinists, are unable to recognise the error of their ways. She is only concerned with 'if': 'If we believe they are unable to recognise that their values are mistaken, we do not hold them responsible for actions that flow from these values...'(p.50). She did not inquire why some people overcome or rebel against what they see as mistaken beliefs or values in their upbringing or environment. It is as important, for example, to know that not all children who are abused go on to abuse others as it is to know that most adults who abuse were abused as children. In Wolf's view it can only be assumed that those who do not abuse had the ability to question this, act on their questioning and are thus sane. Those who do not question, and do not change, lack this ability and, according to Wolf, are not sane. It would also seem to imply that those who question but decide not to change, because, for example, they enjoy abusing, also lack something and are therefore not sane.

This does not seem to be helpful in looking at responsibility in people with a mental illness. Abusers would not generally be described as mentally ill, nor would slave owners, Nazis or male chauvinists. The gulf between insanity, as defined by Wolf, and mental illness seems too wide to make the sane deep-self useful in defining responsibility in people who have a mental illness. In her defence, Wolf was interested in the metaphysics of responsibility and not practical clinical decisions. She could thus argue that the impossible requirement for responsibility, that to be responsible the responsible person has to create themselves, 'turns out to be the vastly more mundane and non-controversial requirement that the responsible agent must, in a fairly standard sense, be sane' (p.47).

The problem with arguing the legal definition of sanity is that it focuses on moral understanding and responsibility and the need for a crime to have been committed. It does not assist questioning whether the mad can be responsible in a non-moral sense, for example cognitively or emotionally in not recognising or understanding how their actions will affect them or others. Responsibility here is contrasted with moral responsibility in the sense of duty to themselves and others. They might hold unusual beliefs which do not lead them to conform socially, lead them to live on the fringe of society but also not do anything else which brings into question their moral responsibility. Neither does it always help in considering civil commitment and control where no crime has taken place.

A problem arises if having an insane deep-self implies that people with mental illness are not responsible for all their actions, or even all their actions which have a moral aspect. It puts both the sane and insane in an impossible position in respect of their everyday lives. Is there anything the insane can make decisions about and be responsible for? If, however, sanity is a normative term, then it would be possible to argue that where their beliefs, behaviours and values conform to the wider society we can label them sane, and thus responsible, and it is only when their beliefs, behaviours and values do not correspond to the 'real world view' they are held to be insane and thus not responsible. The dangers inherent in simply equating sanity with social conformity are evident through political and other abuse but outwith the scope of this book.

Wolf's view also seemed to end up misrepresenting the M'Naghten Rules (where she started). Whereas Wolf confers non-responsibility on a wider range of people than might be considered usual, the M'Naghten Rules serve to limit, severely, those amongst the mad and mentally ill who are legally insane and thus not responsible.

In his account of moral responsibility, Wallace (1994) gave a central place to 'distinctly rational powers'. Arguing from a compatibilist position he asserted that freedom of will is less the issue than 'a form of normative competence; the ability to grasp and apply moral reasons, and to govern one's behaviour by the light of such reasons' (p.1). This led him to assert that to establish what it means to be a morally responsible agent involves understanding what it means to hold someone responsible, and also to investigate the principle of fairness.

Wallace brought together two separate strands of philosophy which he suggested have been treated separately until now; namely a Strawsonian strand derived from *Freedom and Resentment* and the Kantian approach outlined in *Religion within the Limits of Reason Alone*. The Strawsonian position involves understanding responsibility within 'the reactive attitudes' or the range of attitudes which impact on how we behave to each other. The Kantian position requires moral agency which involves the individual being able to consider their desires and goals in relation to moral principles. Combining these ideas he proposed that it is possession of the powers of reflective self-control which is central to moral responsibility and what makes it fair to hold people responsible. It is also what is lacking in those people who are not held responsible.

Wallace described two ways in which a person may not be held responsible: excuses and exemptions. Excuses make it inappropriate to hold an essentially ordinary agent responsible for a particular act and thus apply to the action and not the person. Exemptions, on the other hand, apply to the person and make it inappropriate to hold them responsible in general. Following Strawson, Wallace described two sub-groups of exemptions. Conditions are time-limited and cover conditions such as hypnotism, extreme stress or physical deprivation and the short-term effects of certain drugs. Then there are the 'more systematic and persistent states' (p.155) in which the person's '*normal* condition' (my italics) is such that it would be unfair to hold them morally responsible. These states would include 'insanity or mental illness, extreme youth, psychopathy, and the effects of systematic behaviour control or conditioning' (p.155). This is an interesting list, mixing together as it does internal and external factors.

Wallace suggested that mental illness is a legitimate exemption because it is 'believed to interfere with the powers of reflective self-control' (p.162). Using the M'Naghten Rules to illustrate his point Wallace argued for a 'defect of reason' that prevents the person accurately assessing their moral act because they are deprived of the powers of reflective self-control. Thus, even 'if the agent retains the ability to grasp the moral principles we hold her to, she will lack the ability to apply them correctly in the situations she actually confronts' (p.169).

Although Wallace included mental illness as a 'persistent state' exemption, he did allow that it may, in fact, be a transient state applying to only part of the person's capacity to make moral decisions. Wallace concluded that there are situations, therefore, in which it is fair to hold someone who is mentally ill morally responsible. These would be, for example, decisions taken outside a delusional system which was depriving the person of the power of reflective self-control in a proscribed area.

This is a particularly important point since it should require us to be clear about which aspects of a person with mental illness's behaviour are deemed outwith their control, and thus for which they are not responsible, and those parts for which it is assumed they still retain responsibility. The criminal law sets this out in a way which the civil law does not.

The relationship between the judge and the judged

The decision to label someone mentally ill is an external judgement which may or may not be accepted by the person so judged. Indeed, it is in the cases where it is not accepted that mental health legislation comes into play. If the person accepts they are ill, complies with treatment and takes on an appropriate 'patient role' they are unlikely to put themselves in a position where it will be necessary to use the powers of a mental health law. They could be defined as 'the responsible mentally ill', not only because they accept they are ill but because they take what is defined as a 'responsible' or appropriate response to their problem. This would not, however, prevent them being held not responsible for some of their actions which are believed to be brought about through illness. An important issue here in defining responsible is how the person relates their present situation to what is likely to happen in the future.

French (1992) suggested the Principle of Responsive Adjustment (PRA) as a way of limiting the response to an event to responsibility. He describes PRA thus: 'Moral responsibility may be assigned specifically because the perpetrator, subsequent to the event, failed to respond to its occurrence with an appropriate modification of the behaviour that had as an outcome the unwanted harmful effects' (p.12).

In other words, if, following a negative event, a person who contributed to that event is expected to take action to prevent a recurrence, and if they do not do so, then that person can be held morally responsible in the future. This does not mean that the person is held to have acted intentionally in the original event, but by failing to change, or adjust, the person associates themself with the earlier event.

This relates to mental health legislation, which manages to cast the two 'sides' (the person with mental illness and the public) as both vulnerable and having a duty to the other. The person with mental illness has a duty to consider the impact of their actions on society as a whole as well as its individual members and to act so as not to harm, at the very least, individual members. Society, meanwhile, has a duty not to act in a way which harms (unnecessarily) people who are mentally ill and whom, in some ways at least, seem to have been absolved of responsibility.

Smiley (1992) discussed responsibility in a framework of social and community relations and suggested that in order to understand moral responsibility it needs to be seen in the context of blameworthiness. She thus placed it in a utilitarian framework of Mill (1861/1969) rather than that of Kantian free will. This meant seeing causal responsibility not simply as factual, but as a relationship between an individual, an external state of affairs and a judge or adjudicator. She suggested that rarely do we take into account our role in ascribing blame or not. This is important in mental illness since it could be argued that it is society's role in allowing only some conditions to fall within the remit of mental health legislation that is as important in deciding whether someone is held responsible or not as the actions of individuals themselves. This seems to relate to some 'factual' judgement of responsibility; people who are psychotic cannot be held responsible (in its broadest sense, including cognitively, rather than a more narrow moral sense) whereas people who are neurotic or are addicted to drugs can.

This would seem to rest, to some extent, on society's ability to control the person's 'psychological processes', with answers sought from science and cultural beliefs about 'where to draw the line on self-indulgence' (p.229). Smiley argued that the 'plea of insanity' is accepted as a 'valid excuse' because it is also accepted that the will of insane people is not free.

The role of blaming serves to regulate, possibly undermine, social and personal relationships by creating divisions, especially where blame threatens to exclude the blamed from society. Suggesting that some form of blaming cannot be eliminated altogether, Smiley pointed out that toleration presupposes blame and also the dangers of oppressive supportiveness.

This latter point might be seen in relation to people with mental illness. The very explanation which excuses responsibility and excites support, if not toleration, is also felt by those so excused as oppression. The difficulty here is that whereas a person may reject blame, claiming their actions were not wrong, that the standards set are too high, and that if they have sufficient power or credibility they may persuade others to their point of view, to reject an excuse for not being blamed is more difficult. In some cases it may be possible to argue against unreasonable expectations of behaviour but in others, to argue against the 'excuse', illness, is to accept full moral responsibility.

This has important implications for how an individual with mental illness is judged in relation to their adherence to treatment, especially medication. A first psychotic episode may bring with it a variety of antisocial, disruptive behaviours which everyone who comes in contact with the patient agrees are part of the illness. As a first episode such behaviour had not been predicted, but the behaviour responds to medication. There are five broad categories of response by an individual to this situation:

1. Fiona accepts that she is ill, takes the medication, does well on it and has few relapses. She has some side-effects but maintains medication even when she starts to become ill.

2. Mhairi does not take the medication because she does not believe she is ill. She relapses and can only be treated under the Mental Health Act. She never voluntarily agrees to take medication or enter hospital and hates psychiatrists and other mental health professionals whom she believes are plotting against her.

3. Fraser agrees that he is ill but does not agree to take medication because of unpleasant and severe side-effects. These have affected his personal relationships. He feels that the quality of his life on medication is not worth living and would rather risk periods of acute illness.

4. Bruce accepts that he is ill and despite side-effects takes his medication most of the time. When he starts to relapse he is unlikely to accept that he is becoming ill, question whether he is ill at all and stop his medication. This hastens his relapse.

5. Ewan does not believe he is ill and hates psychiatrists, other mental health professionals and the police, all of whom he believes are plotting against him. He has observed, however, that if he takes his medication regularly these people are much more likely to leave him alone, he is less likely to be taken into hospital against his will and his life is generally quieter and more pleasant. He reluctantly takes his medication, but achieves a life with little interference.

If any of these five people commit an act with negative outcomes while ill are they, or should they, be treated differently?

It might be argued that Fraser is more responsible than the rest since he has accepted that he is ill but refuses to do anything about it or, more specifically, refuses to take medication because of the negative effects to himself. If, in thus preserving his own quality of life, he seriously adversely affects another, this might be viewed as unfair and he is held responsible. If, however, rather than harming others it is himself he harms when he becomes ill is the response the same? His argument here might be that the 'good' (in relative terms) times are paid for with the 'bad' times, but that the trade off is worth it. If it is agreed that he is responsible since he has chosen not to take preventative action, might it then be questioned why he could still be treated under a mental health Act rather than being treated as any other person who does not prevent untoward events, using the criminal law where appropriate or leaving that person to sort out their own mess? The problem is, of course, when he is acutely ill he might then be deemed incapable of taking responsibility while in the state into which he has allowed himself to drift.

Generally civil mental health legislation does not consider responsibility and the aim is to prevent harm, to the person themself and to others. Such legislation seems to accept mental illness as a global exemption, not just for responsibility, but also for allowing people to make choices which may have negative outcomes. If it is assumed that it is 'fair' not to hold those with a mental illness responsible for any of their actions connected with the illness, or while they are ill, this is a much wider concept of non-responsibility than that found under either British, European, or American law in terms of criminal insanity and responsibility.

Extended responsibility and mental illness

When something goes wrong and there is a negative event it seems natural that people look for someone whom they can hold responsible and who can be blamed. When the person who has caused the negative event is deemed not responsible because they have a mental illness there is a void; the chain of events is understood but blame is still missing. If part of the purpose of attaching responsibility is to change the future then there is a problem in effecting this change. In such circumstances it seems that the net of responsibility is cast wider, to the professionals who were treating (or should have treated) the person, particularly the psychiatrist. Even in cases where the family is still held 'responsible' for causing the mental condition it is unlikely that people expect the family to prevent or control the ill person's behaviour.

The psychiatrist can be seen as responsible in two ways. First, they are the person who has diagnosed the perpetrator as having a mental illness and thus removed them from the legitimate realm of the blameworthy. Second, it is perceived that they have the power to control the person, to bring about change in the ill person's behaviour, through treatment (most commonly medication) and thus, potentially, to prevent the negative act.

If something goes wrong and it is discovered that the person with mental illness was not taking their medication then there are two options: first, to blame the person for not taking it, and second, to blame the psychiatrist for not making sure the person takes their medication.

Managing this problem, and apportioning blame, has been part of the review of the Mental Health Act in England and Wales. The government sought to place responsibility on both parties. It argued that patients had a responsibility to take their medication and placed the responsibility for ensuring that patients do so and are not a danger to the public on psychiatrists (Atkinson 2006).

Within such a framework advance directives can be seen as an exercise in taking responsibility for what happens in the future and might thus have been expected to be embraced more warmly by the government than they were. This might reflect a prevailing anxiety that people are more likely to want to opt out of treatment than opt in. It does not, however, deal with the question of the relationship between the well and ill person and whether the well person can, or should, make decisions binding on the ill person.

PART III

Advance Directives in Practice

CHAPTER 10

Advance Directives and the Research Process

Before considering the research evidence for making advance directives, their impact and the experience of using them a few comments must be made about the problems of conducting research in this area, including the actual research questions asked and the methodology employed.

Carrying out research on any aspect of mental health legislation – and psychiatric advance directives can be seen as part of this – is fraught with problems which have been described in detail elsewhere (Atkinson *et al.* 2005; Dawson *et al.* 2001). People cannot be deprived of their legal rights and safeguards or escape mandatory sanctions to fulfil the requirements of a research protocol, such as a randomised controlled trial (RCT). This leads, therefore, to a preponderance of naturalistic or descriptive studies which often do not provide the kind of clear answer for which people are looking. An example of this is in looking at the success, or otherwise, of community treatment orders. Even where two research teams in the USA managed the impressive feat of getting legal permission and support for their trials (Steadman *et al.* 2001; Swartz and Swanson 2004) there were still many limitations to their work. There is a difference, however, in managing legal sanctions, such as compulsory treatment, and voluntarily chosen options such as advance directives.

The longer history of advance directives in the USA means that more research comes from there. A major research project was launched at Duke University, North Carolina in September 2003 with an award of US$1.98 million from the National Institute of Mental Health along with additional money from the MacArthur Foundation and the Greenwall Foundation (Duke University 2003). This study will involve more than 500 patients who have a serious psychiatric disorder. A major focus is to consider the impact of having a trained facilitator in assisting the making of the advance directive.

Caution must always be applied when extrapolating research findings from one country to another. Differences in the organisation of health care will necessarily have an impact, not least between privately insured health care and systems such as the National Health Service (NHS). With respect to advance directives the particular legislation involved will clearly be a major factor in the research findings. In the USA advance directives in mental health usually include the opportunity to appoint a proxy decision-maker of some type for health care, but not in Britain. Written advance directives (instructions) of a person's wishes and appointing a proxy may be seen as very different things by many people, but most of the American research does not separate these two approaches. This means that much of the evidence from the USA may have limited relevance to legal jurisdictions where advance directives do not include appointing proxies. On the other hand, there are likely to be many commonalities in the practicalities of making them.

The purpose of psychiatric advance directives

A basic question might be 'Do advance directives work?' This requires a number of supplementary questions, or at least issues raised, for it to make sense. 'Work' has multiple meanings in this context.

A fundamental issue is how the advance directive is seen, and what is its purpose? Whether it is seen primarily as a tool to promote autonomy or foster co-operation and communication will determine what sort of outcome is expected and thus what to measure. Thus in the first case, the patient feeling that their wishes were respected, regardless of clinical outcome, or whether the outcome was what was anticipated, might be the most important variable. In the second case the variables which are important might have to do with agreement, joint decisions and preventing conflict. Whether psychiatric advance directives 'work' will therefore depend on an understanding of what they are expected to do.

If the professionals involved in the clinical (rather than research) aspects of the study do not take advance directives seriously then this may well affect not only whether patients want to sign up to advance directives (Thomas 2003) but also their effectiveness. In the study by Papageorgiou *et al.* (2002), for example, it was clear that the staff's awareness of the advance directive was limited.

Where advance directives are used with no clear philosophical or value orientation or where they have been introduced through legislation which allows them to develop variably, or those involved to have different (and possibly opposing) views, then the outcome chosen may not be important to all those involved. This leads naturally to ask whose perspective is being considered.

Perspective

A patient who was not compelled to take medication they did not want may count the advance directive a success, even if they spent more time in hospital than they would if they had taken medication. The patient's doctor, however, may have a different view, if they believe the patient could, and should, have been treated. Nursing staff who have to care for patients on the ward may experience difficulties in caring for (increasing numbers of) such patients and present yet a different view. Still further, the patient's family will have a view which may or may not accord with that of the patient. Where a patient refuses treatment through an advance directive, but is not hospitalised, and the family is left to cope with potentially disruptive behaviour, their view may be particularly important and may depend on whether they had input into the advance directive. It may not just be the impact on them as carers which is of concern. Where someone has an advance directive where the outcome might lead to death the family may believe they have a right to have their views considered.

One approach to the research would be to look at multiple perspectives and to triangulate these as appropriate. It is also necessary to understand the range of impacts or outcomes. It is likely that similar consequences may have different impacts on patients, or be viewed differently. Not least in contributing to this will be unintended consequences.

Unintended consequences

People will make an advance directive with certain consequences in mind. Another approach to outcomes would be to ask patients when they make an advance directive what they hope, or intend, the outcome to be and compare their views with what actually happened. This would be helpful in dealing with the problem of unintended consequences. Thus a patient who finds themselves involuntarily hospitalised (but not treated) as a consequence of refusing treatment, and who had not anticipated this, may feel cheated of their sense of autonomy. Someone whose period of untreated illness stretched into months or years rather than the anticipated weeks may feel the loss of time was not compensated for by the sense of autonomy. The person who chooses to opt into treatment may discover that their views over what triggers this differ to what actually happened, to their subsequent consternation.

Other 'unintended consequences' may, in fact, be predicted by those who do not make the advance directive. Concern has already been expressed that people may spend long periods in hospital without treatment, turning hospitals into 'warehouses' (Appelbaum 2004) or put pressure on beds (Halpern and Szmukler 1997). This may place an unacceptable pressure on services and beds for voluntary patients and those who agree or take medication or other treatments.

Clinical outcomes

Much of the research uses clinical outcomes to measure the success of advance directives. How appropriate is this?

Advance directives are not a 'treatment' and may not even be a method of delivering a treatment or a service. Thus to look at days in hospital or relapse or use of mental health legislation with no reference to what the patient intended by the advance directive may be somewhat perverse if the conclusion is that they do not work (because, for example, they did not prevent relapse) but that is not what was intended. This is not to say that such information may not be useful to service providers in planning, or as information for people wanting to make advance directives, but it is unlikely to be measuring their core purpose.

Another problem with taking an overly clinical or treatment approach to advance directives is losing what some see as the core purpose – the patient's choice, to make one as well as its contents. This will affect methodology. How useful is it to compare outcomes between those with and without advance directives when in practice these will be two different groups of people? Similarly, in a randomised research trial it would either mean that some patients who wanted an advance directive did not get one, or some patients who did not want one were 'encouraged' to make one, but with little clinical commitment. In either case this does not mirror clinical practice.

Other objections to the use of randomisation are raised by Thomas and Cahill (2004) who questioned its appropriateness in complex social interventions which are dependent on contextual factors, where it is difficult to specify clearly the 'active components', all of which makes replication problematic.

Even supposing those with an advance directive did 'better' on some clinical outcome, leading an advance directive to be seen as a useful adjunct to treatment regimes, to put patients in a position where they had (or felt they had) to make one would defeat the purpose of advance directives being a statement of choice or self-determination. An explanation of why people were not interested, however, which then addressed these problems, especially where they had to do with institutional barriers, might be more helpful.

Recruitment into such studies is likely to be carried out more enthusiastically than in everyday clinical situations and thus uptake needs to be considered from naturalistic as well as research settings. This also raises questions about reporting uptake. Should the total population or eligible population be used? If the making of an advance directive is an option (or a right) extended to all capacitous patients then maybe this population should be used. Thus patients who cannot be traced, or do not speak English or whatever else excludes them from research, should be included in the denominator. This might show that a substantial number of people are being excluded from studies, but who might wish to avail themselves of the opportunity if presented. It could be argued, for example, that where language is a problem there is an even greater need for an advance directive. It might also be useful to know the size of the group excluded for reasons of mental incapacity.

Whether reporting clinical outcomes should follow an intention to treat model is debatable. Though it could be useful for predicting their impact if used by groups of patients, it runs the risk of turning what should be a matter of individual choice into another expectation put on patients or a hoop through which they must jump.

Lastly Amering, Stastny and Hopper (2005) made the point that patients may need to work at their own pace in initiating an advance directive. This is rarely allowed for in research trials and may be reflected in less than positive outcomes, particularly around uptake.

At this stage it may be most prudent to suggest that a variety of orientations to research methods is likely to have the most useful results.

CHAPTER 11

Making and Implementing
Advance Directives
in Mental Health

This chapter looks at the various stages of advance directives and the practical issues involved in making and implementing them and draws on the limited research in the area. Chapter 12 looks at how various types of directive work in practice. A note of caution should be applied to extrapolating directly from the research into practice, in that research studies often have more resources, particularly staff time, available for the setting up of the directives.

There are three main stages in the management of advance directives in practice:

• making an advance directive

• invoking an advance directive

• reviewing and changing an advance directive.

Making an advance directive
The process of making an advance directive may be broken down into a number of stages which can be framed as practical questions.

• Who can (or should) make an advance directive?

• When should it be made?

• How should it be made?

• What should it contain?

• Who should witness it?

• How and where should it be stored?

Who can (or should) make an advance directive?

Although the simplest answer to this might be 'anyone' who has capacity, the literature (and possibly common sense) indicates that this is neither the general assumption nor practice. Overwhelmingly the expectation is that a psychiatric advance directive will be made only by (or is only appropriate for) people who have experienced a major mental illness, e.g. Papageorgiou *et al.* (2002), Srebnik *et al.* (2005). Where the advance directive is closer to a joint crisis plan then, by definition, it can only be made by someone who has been ill and is still in touch with services (Henderson *et al.* 2004).

It makes sense that it should be this group of people. They are the group most likely to have an acute episode in the future and therefore the most likely to find an advance directive useful and to have a very good idea of what to expect. In practical terms they are also immediately accessible and this makes introducing and planning the advance directive (not to mention research) easier.

Asking 'Who can make an advance statement?' the Scottish Executive offered a wider view (although elsewhere it implicitly assumes that it will apply only to people who have been ill). Introducing the new advance statements it said:

> If you can understand what you are putting in the statement and the effect it might have on your future treatment, you can make an advance statement.

> This includes young people under 16 years of age so long as you can understand the nature and possible consequences of the procedure or treatment.

> You can make a statement if you are receiving treatment for a mental disorder (mental illness including dementia, learning disability or personality disorder) now, have had treatment in the past, or have never had treatment (Scottish Executive 2004, p.7).

This went further than the proposals by the Millan Committee (Scottish Executive 2001) when reviewing the previous Act (Mental Health Act 1984) in preparation for the new Act, who simply said, 'Service users should be entitled to make advance statements...'

The main criterion for someone making an advance statement is that they are competent. The issues surrounding this have been dealt with in Chapter 5. There is no absolute standard for assessing competency to make an advance statement, although there is some work addressing this issue (Srebnik, Appelbaum and Russo 2004). This is described in the next chapter.

Unless psychiatric advance directives are specifically defined/legislated to be made in conjunction with mental health staff (and are thus advance agreements, joint crisis plans or similar) it would seem reasonable to suggest that anyone can make one. The question of how informed the decisions are, however, is likely to be raised at the time of activation. Electro-convulsive therapy (ECT), for example, may be refused by a patient (who has not had it before), supported by relatives, even as a final resort. The reasoning is usually based on negative media stories. The problem is exacerbated when people do not realise the potentially life-threatening implications of some conditions. Unlike end-of-life situations, which people may be able to imagine even from a young(ish) age (or, indeed, encouraged to consider in organ donor campaigns), few people are likely to envisage developing a major mental illness and losing capacity. And since most people will not be in this position, promoting advance directives for mental illness is unlikely to be appropriate. One group, however, who might have more interest are those people who are at high risk of developing a major mental illness, probably through a genetic link.

Advance directives may also be of particular use for people with poor English (or other verbal communication problems), in that they make clear the person's intentions. Where interpreting services are slow to respond this may save considerable confusion, distress and frustration. It has also been pointed out that an advance directive is useful where the clinician's English language skills are poor (Honberg 2000).

When should an advance directive be made?
Beyond the obvious answer of when the person has mental capacity there is little clarity, or indeed evidence, about when an advance directive should be made. The two randomised controlled trials in London differed. Papageorgiou *et al.* (2002) recruited patients coming to the end of a period of compulsory treatment under the Mental Health Act 1983. Henderson *et al.* (2004), discussing joint crisis plans, recruited patients through a local community mental health team and explicitly avoided those who were currently inpatients 'to avoid any coercion to participate'. This was the same timing used by Srebnik *et al.* (2003). Across the research studies the types of advance directives on offer and recruitment strategies used differed so much that comparisons are difficult.

Common sense would suggest that the best time might be when the patient is receptive to a general consideration of the future, including future treatment. For some this might follow on from a relapse or hospitalisation. For others contemplation of another episode in the future at such a time is just too painful. While some might see planning for future episodes as a positive step in gaining some control over what happens, others may see this as 'giving in' to a medically based philosophy or model which is designed to keep them ill.

Although in some ways the patient's psychiatrist is best placed to decide when to introduce the idea, this depends on the psychiatrist believing an advance directive is worthwhile. Since there is some evidence that many psychiatrists do not fully support advance directives, the suggestion may never be made. Probably as important as when it is introduced is someone having the responsibility/duty to bring the option to the patient's attention and facilitate making the directive. This offer may need to be made on more than one occasion. It should not be left solely to patients to raise making an advance directive. The role of the psychiatric nurse in advance directives also needs to be considered (Vuckovich 2003).

Another factor not considered in the research was language. Where it is mentioned in research studies it was as a requirement for patients to be able to read and/or converse in English as an entry criterion. It would be useful to investigate whether poor English makes people more or less likely to want to make an advance directive. Although for people with poor English the advantages may seem clear, having their views clearly expressed in English for other people to read, with no delay in finding an interpreter in a crisis, the reality may not be so straightforward. People who have poor English as a second language may do so for a variety of reasons, including being recent immigrants, which will include asylum seekers and refugees. Living in disadvantaged minority ethnic communities may make people uneasy with what seem to be 'official' forms which require their signature and witnesses. Working with local organisations or charities which support such groups may be particularly important.

The Scottish Executive (2004) gave clear guidance for people for whom English is a second language to seek interpretation and translation support from either their health board or local authority. They pointed out that these organisations have a statutory duty to provide this under the Race Relations (Amendment) Act 2000.

In some minority ethnic or social groups the expectation for autonomous, individual decisions is not the norm and decisions are more likely to be family or group based. This should not preclude someone from making an advance directive, although a format which allows for a co-operative decision to be made with the family may be more appropriate.

How should an advance directive be made?

One of the main considerations here is whether the person makes it independently or with members of their treatment team or other professionals who might influence the decision. Again, there is unlikely to be a one-size-fits-all answer. For some patients an independently made advance directive (and if possible legally enforceable one) will be the only alternative which will satisfy their need to demonstrate autonomy. Other patients may prefer a jointly agreed alternative possibly in the belief that this is more likely to be adhered to.

In a study on crisis cards (Sutherby *et al.* 1999) an interesting outcome occurred. Although able to complete an independent crisis card, all 40 patients who completed a card chose a joint rather than an independent card. This included one card where a disagreement over ECT (the patient wanted to refuse this against advice) was recorded in the joint card, the patient preferring this to an independent card.

The interest, or maybe commitment, of staff seems to be crucial. Where case managers introduced advance directives to patients, having a case manager who supported the advance directive was associated significantly with the patient's interest in making an advance directive (Srebnik *et al.* 2003).

This reinforced an observation made several years earlier by Backlar and McFarland (1996) in a questionnaire study on the use of advance directives. Although there were responses from five psychologists with a total of 14 clients with an advance directive, these all came from the clients of one person. This psychologist noted that, of their 22 clients, 14 (64%) had made an advance directive.

A benefit of making the advance directive with a member of staff is not only about agreement but may also be of considerable importance for patients who have poor literary skills. As well as giving patients an opportunity to talk through what they want and do not want to happen it may assist in wording the advance directive unambiguously or ensure that it conveys exactly what the person intends. All this may improve the advance directive's chances of being followed rather than overturned by a psychiatrist or others concerned about its validity.

Yet another advantage of including a professional, at least in the discussion of content, is that alternatives or resources might be suggested of which the patient was unaware.

The study of joint crisis plans (Henderson *et al.* 2004) involved a number of people in the meeting to make the plan, possibly reflecting the orientation of this type of advance directive (Sutherby, Henderson and Flood 2004). It was suggested that as well as an independent facilitator, 'wherever possible', the meeting should also be attended by the key worker and doctor as well as the patient and anyone the user feels would be useful, 'such as friend, relative or formal advocate'. This meeting of up to five people would follow a preliminary meeting with the key worker to give the user 'a menu'. The average time taken for this meeting was 50 minutes, but it was thought this could be reduced to 30 minutes if all of the basic sections were completed at the preliminary meeting.

All this clearly takes up staff time. In research studies this may not be such an issue if additional research staff are used. In over-stretched mental health services, however, this may prove more problematic. Unless systematically offered to everyone it might result in the more assertive, active or articulate patients receiving support at the expense of others whose need may be even greater. If, however, an outcome study indicated that people with an advance directive made less use of resources (because, for example, their relapses were better managed) than previously, or than those without, it could be argued that involving staff in making them is cost-effective. This is, however, a very limited approach to outcome.

On a purely practical note Srebnik and Brodoff (2003) asked who should be billed for helping a patient make an advance directive. Although this is intended to apply to insurance-led services, even in state-funded services such as the National Health Service (NHS) clarity might be required in terms of job descriptions as to whether this is part of someone's job or not. Time spent on this is time not doing some other task. This would not be the case if it were routine under a general future planning role or if it is simply seen as part of good practice. There is some suggestion that the low uptake of advance statements in Scotland, although provided for in the new mental health law, is because no professional group has a duty or responsibility under the Act to introduce them to patients.

In relation to making advance directives with older people, Schirm and Stachel (1996) suggested that it might be possible to treat the discussions needed to make the directive, in this example as a values history, as counselling and thus billed as such to insurance companies. As more evidence becomes available on the benefits of advance directives it may make clinicians and service managers (as well as insurance companies) more willing to see working with a patient to develop this as a useful endeavour rather than a luxury.

A way around the potential problem of staff time is to develop other methods to give information and support in making an advance directive, for example a computer program. One such program was devised and tested in Colorado by Sherman (1998). The AD-Maker program consisted of four main sections:

- how to use the computer including the mouse (no keyboard was available)

- an interactive, didactic presentation outlining what an advance directive is and related topics

- a basic competency test – this was a true–false comprehension test of the material presented

- an interview section to obtain information to be printed in the advance directive.

A very particular approach was given to the help provided in making the advance directive: 'The program incorporates a strict advocacy approach...for many of the choice points faced by the user there was agreement from the advisory group as to the clear self-advice choice(s), but there were no 'default' answers – users always had to make an active choice' (p.353).

The program itself was multimedia, incorporating sound, pictures and video clips and was designed to run on commonly available hardware. Those chosen to test the program were recruited from two clubhouses and had to meet 'Colorado's …highest priority population (…combinations of certain diagnoses, duration and a minimum level of functional impairment)' (p.354). One-third of those approached declined to take part, with 60 taking part in the program testing. Of these, 37 per cent had a diagnosis of schizophrenia, 22 per cent depression and 13 per cent bipolar disorder. The majority, 36 (60%) had no experience with computers. Of the 60 participants 39 (65%) were able to complete the advance directive in the allocated time. Six (10%) people were unable to pass the comprehension test. Five (8%) stopped before completing the advance directive and 9 (15% ran out of time (approximately 80 minutes). The actual mean time spent was 63 minutes.

The views of users testing the program were overwhelmingly positive with at least 75 per cent reporting favourably on all but one item. Having a menu to choose from was found helpful by everyone: 96 per cent endorsed they were 'able to make more progress in creating my advance directive' using the computer than if 'someone had just given me a blank form to fill in'. It would be recommended to others by 91 per cent, and 88 per cent wanted to use the computer to make an advance directive. People found using the computer 'pleasant and educational' (96%) and found it made them 'feel good' about themselves (80%). The only criticism was that a substantial number wanted to cover things in their advance directive which were not in the program.

The only significant demographic factors linked to being able to complete an advance directive were: ethnicity and learning disability reduced completion rates while having a higher level of education increased completion. No other factors, including diagnosis or presence of hand tremor, were significant.

The AD-Maker program has been used elsewhere with success to enable patients to make advance directives. Srebnik et al. (2005) used it with groups of up to six people at a time, using laptops, led by a peer trainer. This person provided 'an overview of instruction, the documents' legal status, and potential benefits and challenges to their use'.

A low-tech alternative was the 'Preferences of Care' booklet used by Papageorgiou et al. (2002, 2004). Patients completed a series of seven statements. Only five were about what they wanted or did not want to happen and two described what happens when they become ill. There was a limit to what could be written as under each statement there was only space for three entries (Papageorgiou et al. 2004).

In Scotland there is no requirement for the advance statement to be in any particular form. The Scottish Executive's (2004) advice makes the practical point that, although it need not be typed, 'it must be written clearly enough to be read by those who will be caring for you'. A suggested form is given, but the only two areas given are: 'I would like to receive the following treatments' and 'I would *not* like to receive the following treatments'.

Not all laws require an advance directive to be written down, and some will accept an oral directive. It is, however, much more difficult to demonstrate the existence of an oral directive, be clear about what it contains or its validity in terms of the person's competence when making it. Medical records or nursing notes may contain references to conversations or detail consistent decisions, such as refusal of, or preference for, certain treatments, which may be used as evidence for supporting a verbal directive (Derbyshire Mental Health Services NHS Trust 2003).

What should an advance directive contain?

Leaving aside the discussion about opting into or out of treatment, which has been covered earlier, the central issue here is how far an advance directive should extend beyond straightforward treatment choices. Legislation may clarify what is legally sanctioned in a specific jurisdiction.

It should not need stating that an advance directive should start with the person's name and other identifier (such as date of birth, address) so it is clear to whom the directive applies. This, of course, raises issues of privacy and confidentiality should it get lost or inappropriately circulated. This will need addressing with the user if they keep a copy at home and also in respect of copies given to family or friends. Papageorgiou *et al.* (2004) noted that the Preferences of Care booklet had the hospital's name and address printed in it in case the booklet was lost.

Other sections probably follow:

- treatment I want to receive
- treatment I do *not* want to receive
- people to contact
- current clinical support.

People need to give consent for their inclusion if they are being named as someone who will be involved, for example, as a proxy decision-maker or simply someone to support the patient. It is not clear, however, whether this is necessary if it is simply to inform the person of the patient's whereabouts. Thus a patient might want to let a relative or employer know where they are, without this putting any obligation on that person. It would be standard practice in any setting where someone has an emergency admission to hospital to ask who they want to be informed that they have been admitted. Generally, however, the expectation would be that the hospital would contact one person who would then inform others.

In some cases special discretion might need to be exercised. Not everyone might want to be contacted and may have severed ties with the patient. In such circumstances they might experience this as a form of continued harassment. Another group over whom concern has been expressed are people known/ strongly suspected of supplying the patient with illegal drugs, if this were to give them access to the person in hospital.

Clinical support need not be an extensive list but should probably, as a limit, be the patient's psychiatrist and key worker. It should not be assumed that the advance directive will only be activated in the 'home (or local) setting'. Patients who have advance directives might be advised to take a copy with them when they travel, for example on holiday, so as to be prepared for any emergency.

In Scotland the Mental Health (Care and Treatment) (Scotland) Act 2003 clearly states that an advance statement is for how the person wants to be treated, or not treated, if they become ill in the future. Although the law does not specify treatment in terms of therapeutic intervention the Guide provided by the Scottish Executive (2004) and the Code of Practice (Scottish Executive 2005) both make it clear that this is what is intended. The Guide, for example, indicates it is for 'views about medications, therapies or electro-convulsive therapy (ECT)'. Provision is made, however, for people to make an additional 'personal statement'. This is not mentioned in the Act and does not have the same legal standing. It is suggested that this be used to explain whatever else might be important to the person. This could include child or pet care, keeping an employer informed, dietary needs, spiritual life and exercise and relaxation preferences.

It is suggested that where possible reasons are given for treatment decisions which would further aid clinical decisions. The examples given are:

I prefer individual therapy to group therapy because I am uncomfortable with strangers when I am unwell

or

I don't want medications which make me put on weight.

The advice given is thus very general and may not help a person write something which is sufficiently specific nor to think through consequences.

The form provided by Derbyshire Mental Health Services NHS Trust (2003, 2004) has two parts: the first covers treatment and care and the second covers personal and home life, including specific areas for care of pets and the security of the person's home.

In contrast, the AD-Maker had 12 'instruction sections' (Sherman 1998, p.353). These were:

1. a definition of when the AD takes effect and when it is no longer effective;

2. consents and refusals for psychotropic medications;

3. allergies to medications;

4. preferences for medication administration (e.g. oral versus injection and time of day);

5. persons to be immediately notified of an involuntary commitment;

6. persons prohibited from visiting;

7. consent to obtain previous medical records;

8. preferences for hospitals and alternatives to hospital;

9. consents/refusals for ECT;

10. suggestions for how to avert an impending emergency;

11. preferences for emergency psychiatric treatments (i.e. seclusion and restraint);

12. preferences for life-sustaining treatments.

These choices were made from a menu. Even with a list this comprehensive some people still had topics which were not covered but which they wanted to include.

This list was modified in the version used by Srebnik *et al.* (2005) to five treatment and five non-treatment areas. The treatment areas covered 'psychotropic medication, hospital preferences, alternatives to hospitalisation, emergency de-escalation methods..., and ECT' (p.593). The reasons for the preferences were also indicated from a list of options. Users were not allowed to opt out of emergency de-escalation methods entirely and were required to 'rank-order preferences among seclusion, seclusion plus restraint and sedating medication'. Although it was possible to refuse all psychotropic medication the program in fact discouraged this 'by flashing the response option that permitting some psychotropic medication was preferable'.

The five non-treatment or 'personal care' areas were 'persons to notify during hospitalisation, assistive devices to retain during hospitalisation, dietary preferences, and persons to contact to take care of finances, dependants and pets during hospitalisation' (p.395). Users were also able to appoint a surrogate decision-maker and add other instructions.

As well as specifying when the advance directive was to be activated there was an opportunity to state whether they wanted the directive to be revocable at any time or only when they were competent.

Details of choices made are given in the next chapter but it would seem that this was a useful approach to assist patients in clarifying their thoughts about which decisions need to be made and why. By not allowing patients to opt out of emergency measures entirely, for example, it may help bring home the reality that in some situations doing nothing is not an option for staff. An important point to note was that the directives made were 'rated as feasible, useful and consistent with practice standards' in at least 95 per cent of cases. The only exceptions were the choices under the heading 'willingness to try medications not listed in the directive' where 13 per cent of patients (14/106) stated they were unwilling to take medications not listed in their directive and two patients gave no instructions.

The Preferences of Care booklet (Papageorgiou *et al.* 2002) included seven statements to be completed by the patient. These were:

1. I notice I am becoming ill again when I...

2. Things that happened just before I was placed on a section and/or started to become ill were...

3. If I do seem to be becoming ill again I would like...

4. I would like you to contact...

5. I wouldn't want...

6. If I have to be admitted to hospital again I would like...

7. In hospital I would like...

Results were only reported in general categories (Papageorgiou *et al.* 2004) so it is difficult to see how specific responses were but some raise questions about their feasibility, for example, what was included under the heading 'Improved human rights' in response to what is wanted on hospital admission? Only allowing three responses may not allow patients to exercise all the choices they would want to make. In terms of the multi-agency care and support many patients experience, three options is likely to be too few.

The joint crisis plans (Henderson *et al.* 2004) offered patients a menu of four sections. These were: contact information, current care and treatment plan, care in a crisis, and practical help in a crisis (Sutherby *et al.* 2004).

Although not perfect these studies did suggest that only a minority of patients might want to make an advance directive. Before this is taken at face value the way in which they are presented and the reasons given for not wanting to make them need careful scrutiny. Most were offered by members of the patient's clinical team, other clinicians or researchers. Some patients may therefore question their independence. What has not been looked at is the promotion of advance directives through user or self-help groups (although a number pro-vide advice and/or templates) and whether this might influence uptake. Other research, however, has suggested the importance of having clinical staff involved.

The interest in advance directives can also be reported as a 'half-full' or 'half-empty' scenario. Srebnik *et al.* (2003) concluded that 'substantial interest in psychiatric advance directives was shown among individuals with serious and persistent mental illness' although in this case 'substantial' was 53 per cent. Less optimistic researchers may have concluded that a substantial number showed no interest.

Who should witness an advance statement?

It is generally expected that an advance statement will be witnessed, although the purpose of this may vary. The main issue will be whether the witness is attesting to the capacity of the person making the advance directive (and how formal this assessment is) or simply that the person did, in fact, make the advance directive. In the case of the latter position any other capable person should be able to witness the signature. Where the witness is attesting to the capacity of the person, however, the law is likely to give a prescribed list of acceptable witnesses. For example, in Scotland the list is:

- a doctor (it could be your general practitioner or responsible medical officer (RMO) or another doctor)

- a registered nurse (it could be your community psychiatric nurse (CPN) or another nurse)

- a solicitor

- a social worker (it could be your mental health officer or another social worker)

- a clinical psychologist

- an occupational therapist, or

- a social service worker, for example a supervisor or manager of a care service. (Scottish Executive 2004, p.8).

The position of the witness is described to the person making the advance statement as: '…confirming that in their opinion you are able to understand what you have written in the statement and the effect it might have on your future treatment' (Scottish Executive 2004, p.8).

This is a fairly limited approach to capacity. There is no clear expression of how such an assessment of understanding be carried out, nor how the different professional groups will approach this in the same way or have had training in assessing capacity for this purpose. It is suggested that the witness might want to discuss the contents, with the implicit reason that this discussion will be used to determine capacity. It is made clear that the witness does not have to be involved in writing the advance statement and, in particular, that they do not have to agree with it. These two points are likely to be important to patients as they emphasise the independent nature of the advance statement. It should also make the position of a professional asked to witness an advance statement more comfortable if the directive goes against what they would advise or see as best practice.

This position is not restricted to Scotland and different organisations have different views as to how clinical staff should handle the signing of an advance directive. One view is that professionals should not witness a statement which they believe they would not be able to uphold or support if it were invoked, the so-called 'conflict of duty' (Scottish Executive 2004). This can cause particular problems for a patient if they are limited in who they can ask to be a witness.

Another position would be that the professional can sign the advance directive but should explain to the patient their position if they do not agree with the directive's contents and would not be able to support it. In some places advice may go so far as to suggest that this be recorded in writing. Thus in Scotland two versions of what the witness may attest to are given. Under the patient's signature the witness must write: 'I hereby certify that I am of the opinion that at the time of making this advance statement [(patient's) name] has the capacity of properly intending the wishes specified in it. Hereby witness his/her signature' (Scottish Executive 2004, p.9). Where there may be a 'conflict of duty' a suggested form of words to add after the above statement is: 'I have stated my views with respect to my perceived risk of future conflict of duty. I hereby witness his/her signature' (Scottish Executive 2004, p.9). As well as the witness's signature their full name, address and date must be added. Where someone feels unable to act as a witness, particularly because of conflict of duty, they should, nevertheless, help the patient to find someone who is able to act as their witness.

A further issue regarding witnesses is that some might require payment, which might limit some patients' access to them. Srebnik and Brodoff (2003) have already raised the issue of billing for time spent in assisting making an advance directive. If an assessment of capacity is part of the witness's duties, no matter how rudimentary, then this will take time. Even within the NHS not everyone may see it as part of their job. General practitioners, for example, expect to be paid for this as it is seen by them as an additional service. Lawyers will also charge for this. Even though financial support through legal aid may be available, for some people this will be an additional bureaucratic form too far.

It is understandable that authorities wanted to ensure that advance directives are witnessed by someone 'appropriate'. Appropriate here might include someone whose own capacity will not be open to question (as it might be if signed by another patient) or who is not bringing pressure to bear on the patient to make a certain set of conditions in their advance directive. This might include family members, friends or others being given access to the person when they would not want it, access to information about them or control of their finances. Where clinicians are involved in making advance agreements or joint plans they will, of course, have a vested interest in the decisions made. It could be argued that such agreements should be witnessed by someone who can attest to the patient's signing the agreement being voluntary or free from coercion. This might be both a difficult responsibility to put on an individual and difficult to verify.

How and where should an advance directive be stored?

The main criteria here is that it should be immediately and easily available to the treating doctor (and possibly others) at the time it needs to be invoked. Ideally it should not rely on a possibly very ill and confused patient reminding people of its existence and place of storage. An advance directive which cannot be accessed at such a time, or which no one knows exists is, literally, not worth the paper it is written on.

In Scotland a fairly extensive list is provided of people to whom a copy of the advance directive should be given. This covers, where they exist:

- named person

- carer

- family

- solicitor

- nurse

- independent advocate

- guardian

- welfare attorney

- responsible medical officer

- mental health officer

- general practitioner

- other people close to you (Scottish Executive 2004, p.10).

There are advantages and disadvantages in such an extensive list. The more people who have a copy the easier it might be to access it when it is needed. It might also help to authenticate it as an up-to-date document. Conversely, the more people who have a copy the more time and effort there is in recalling the advance directive and issuing a new directive should changes be made. Also the more copies in existence the less it might be treated as a confidential document. Although it is to be hoped that professionals, whether clinical staff, lawyers or social services staff, understand its confidential nature and treat it as they would other medical or social care records, this would need to be impressed on family and friends. There is maybe a distinction to be drawn here between a wide range of people knowing that an advance directive exists and where a copy is kept (e.g. medical records at designated hospital/GP surgery/lawyer) and everyone having a copy of the full directive. It may also be important that anything not kept in hospital records, or with a family member, may not be accessible out of hours.

An obvious place to store an advance directive would seem to be at the front of the patient's medical record and it should be expected this would be easily found by staff when needed. That this is not necessarily the case was demonstrated by Papageorgiou *et al.* (2004). The Preferences for Care booklet (size 15cm × 10.5 cm) was given to the patient's key worker and general practitioner and copies placed in hospital and general practice records (Papageorgiou *et al.* 2002). Two of the researchers confirmed that it was at the front of the case notes one year after it had been placed there (Papageorgiou *et al.* 2004). Despite these measures, at one year follow-up few psychiatrists expected to find the Preference for Care booklets useful or even know of their existence.

Whether computerised storage of advance directives would have helped in this case, or elsewhere, has not really been studied. Even where records are computerised there is no guarantee that clinicians will note their presence on screen any more than they do at the front of paper notes. One approach might be to have a computerised record which not only flags up an advance directive at the outset but also requires confirmation that this had been noted. This could be tedious, however, when records are assessed many times without the need to consult the directive because the patient is competent or because it is being followed. It could be amended to require consultation before hospitalisation or before compulsory measures are taken. The latter would put it in the same position as an advance statement in Scotland.

Patients may choose to be proactive and carry their advance directive with them, although this probably assumes a small, discrete document. An alternative may be a type of medical alert bracelet or pendant which states the existence of an advance directive and its location. Although these are routinely used by people with allergies or particular medical conditions, and there is an assumption that they will be automatically noted by medical and nursing staff, this may not always be the case.

No storage system, however, is going to overcome indifference and apathy of clinical staff. It is unreasonable to expect patients who are acutely ill or in crisis to alert staff to the presence of an advance directive. In these circumstances there are three ways forward. One would be to continue to raise awareness of advance directives amongst clinical staff, probably coupled with the second, which is to have the patient's carer or close friend or relative (whoever must be contacted on admission) have a copy, or at least know of the existence and whereabouts of the advance directive. These approaches will be important where the person is not going to be detained under mental health legislation but there may still be concerns about capacity.

Where a person is going to be detained, a third, more formal, approach might be necessary. In Scotland the mental health officer (MHO) has a duty to inquire of the patient, at the time of assessment for detention/compulsory treatment, whether the patient has an advance statement. Anecdotal comments from MHOs who have done this suggest that where a patient is floridly psychotic this is easier said than done. There is, however, a requirement that anyone treating a patient under the Act has to take an advance statement into account. This includes not only the patient's treating doctor but a second opinion doctor who is consulted about the authorisation of some treatments under the Act and also the mental health tribunal where a patient is being assessed for compulsory treatment.

Invoking an advance directive

When to invoke or activate an advance directive is not as straightforward as it might seem at first sight. It must always be remembered that in the eyes of the law a person is presumed to have capacity unless legally declared otherwise, or unless good cause can be shown for presuming otherwise to allow, for example, emergency treatment. Thus invoking an advance directive necessarily means that a judgement about capacity has to be made. How formal this judgement is will depend on a number of factors.

Where there is clear law governing a psychiatric advance directive, whether incorporated into mental health law or as a separate statute, this should indicate when the advance directive is to be activated, even then the position may not be clear-cut. In Scotland, for example, it is clear that once a patient comes under the provisions of the Mental Health (Care and Treatment) (Scotland) Act 2003 account has to be taken of any existing advance statement. One of the criteria for using the Act is that the person has impaired ability to make decisions about their medical treatment. There is, however, the possibility that the person has impaired ability but does not meet the other risk criteria for the Act to be used. It would seem iniquitous if, in such circumstances, an advance directive were not invoked.

In most places with specific legislation for psychiatric advance directives the activation of the advance directive is usually when the patient is unable to take in and evaluate information relating to their medical care, and is thus deemed incapable. This does not always have to be a decision made in court, but requires some combination of one or more physicians, psychiatrists, mental health social workers and court. Where the law allows for a proxy, either through the advance directive or other form of power of attorney (e.g. durable power of attorney, DPOA), there may be provision for the maker of the advance directive to set the time at which the DPOA takes effect (e.g. the state of Washington). Although it would be possible to make it effective immediately it is normally some time in the future which may be linked to a particular time or event. This may not be linked to incapacity as such, but to a more general state of disability. Thus admission to hospital may, in itself, be enough to trigger the power of attorney or it may be linked to an earlier event, such as spending more than a certain amount of money or acting in a way which would put the person's employment or relationships at risk. In some cases it is the person with power of attorney who is able to state when an advance directive is to be invoked.

Where there is no legal determination for invoking an advance directive, similar 'triggering events' might be included in the advance directive. Care has to be taken that advance directives are not simply invoked when a person becomes acutely ill. To do so would be to equate being psychotic or severely depressed with being incompetent, which is an unreasonable assumption. That is not to say that such patients may have difficulty making treatment decisions through some combination of unwillingness, inability, ambivalence, indecision or simply being overwhelmed by the situation. This 'netherworld of quasi competence' as described by Dunlap (2000–1) leads her to suggest that 'a voluntary commitment contract may be available to take effect during that period where incompetence cannot be established but the person may be suffering the ill effects of mental illness nevertheless' (p.355).

Others, including patients, however, may see the activation of the advance directive early in the crisis or acute episode as an important guide to staff as to the care and treatment the patient wants (Ritchie *et al.* 1998). In such cases crisis plan might be a better name. A similar point is made that advance directives can protect someone falling 'through the cracks' when, as they become ill, they disengage from, or do not seek, treatment but who also do not meet the criteria for compulsory treatment (Sales 1993).

This raises again the question of the type and purpose of the advance directive. If they are to provide early treatment (which might be refused) to prevent or de-escalate a crisis and prevent hospitalisation and/or compulsory treatment then the threshold for invoking the advance directive might be 'lower' than where their aim is for the patient to be able to refuse treatment. It might be assumed that psychiatrists or other treating doctors would be more willing to invoke an advance directive that provides for treatment earlier than one which refuses treatment. If, however, a person is refusing treatment and does not meet the legal criteria for compulsory treatment or detention the effect might be the same.

The law tends not to be clear about how and when treatment specified in a psychiatric advance directive can be imposed on a person who is currently refusing (is not capable of changing the advance directive) and who does not meet the requirements for compulsory treatment. Both service providers and courts may prefer to have statutory guidance on this (Srebnik and Brodoff 2003) rather than 'go it alone'.

Advance agreements (or joint crisis plans) may fit better into this arrangement and, by their very name, are designed to deal with crises (which may be specified as certain events, circumstances, behaviours/symptoms) and are triggered then rather than only by incapacity.

The research trials on advance directives are less than illuminating on when they were invoked. The first statement in the Preferences of Care booklet (Papageorgiou *et al.* 2002, 2004) outlines the signs that the patient is becoming ill. The second outlines what happened just before they were put on a section or became ill previously. It is not made clear if these are intended as triggers for consulting the other choices in the booklet. Since the main outcome measured was reduction in involuntary commitment it might appear that it was when this was being considered that the 'directive' would be triggered. The time and process for using the booklet was not clear from the published reports and the low use, and even awareness of it, by psychiatrists might suggest this was not clear to them either.

The joint crisis plan introduced by Henderson *et al.* (2004) also used reduction of compulsory admission or treatment and other admission as its outcome measures. Again no indication of how the plans were invoked is given but the assumption is when these circumstances arise. In neither study is the use of these advance agreements overtly linked to the formal assessment of, or definition of, incapacity.

If there are formal requirements for a capacity assessment before an advance directive is invoked (which may accompany an assessment for detention under mental health legislation) this will limit the use of advance directives. Many psychiatrists appear unwilling to declare a patient incapable unless detention, guardianship or similar circumstances exist. This formal approach to invoking psychiatric advance directives is likely to reduce their use, and thus usefulness in promoting patient choice and autonomy.

Paradoxically, however, their earlier use with a less formal (i.e. legal) assessment of capacity may infringe current choice in circumstances which the patient had not anticipated, or before they had expected them to be used. This may be overcome by patients specifying in their advance directive when it is to be invoked, but again, it is difficult to envisage all situations and circumstances.

This may be further complicated if the advance directive covers more than just medical treatment. Patients may be impaired in making a decision about their clinical care but capable of making other decisions. Although this will only cause practical problems if decisions in the advance directive differ from current decisions it cannot be optimal, or in accordance with the least restrictive alternative, to be using the advance directive where it is not necessary, yet to argue for only invoking parts of it is likely to be problematic.

Revoking and changing a psychiatric advance directive

The main issue here is whether the law allows a person to change or revoke their advance directive at any time or only when they are capacitous. To many it seems odd that a directive, designed to make a person's competent wishes clear, can be changed by that same person when incompetent. It raises the question 'Why bother?' Others see it as a response to either the problem of the relationship between the past and current person or a practical way of reacting to changing circumstances and unpredictable illness episodes. The arguments might be slightly different when opt-in and opt-out directives are considered. It is worth noting that in one study (Swanson *et al.* 2003), although neither patients, clinicians nor family members as groups supported being able to revoke an advance directive when ill, patients were significantly more likely to support this than the other groups (although still in a minority).

Where the person has opted out of (certain) treatment and then changes their mind, clinicians may be happy to accept this, possibly choosing to see it as the beginning of a return to capacity. Even where the person remains incapable it may make all concerned more comfortable in overturning the advance directive. In most cases clinicians are likely to follow patients' choices where they opt for treatment and maintaining and preserving health and life than not.

The legitimacy of such choice, however, might be questioned when it comes not to an active request but more in the form of 'do what you like', or 'I don't care' in a patient worn down by illness and possible pressure from clinicians and family and friends. Views of incapable people are listened to and taken as valid in circumstances where there is no former capacity and no prospect of capacity. Thus people with a degree of learning disability which renders them incapable are, nevertheless, consulted about their care and life as far as is possible. Other changes are allowed. Incompetent patients with a DNR (do not resuscitate) but who indicate they want to live will usually be treated. Women with birth plans who change their mind and want pain relief during labour will receive it.

One area where advance directives are routinely changed by a person who may lack capacity and the change acted on by clinicians is during labour. Birth plans made by pregnant women often request 'natural child birth' and no medication for pain. It is not uncommon, however, for women to change their mind during labour and request pain relief. This is given, and to most people it would be inconceivable for the doctor or midwife to say to the woman, 'Several months ago you said you didn't want pain relief so you're not getting it'. This is despite the fact that everybody understands that pain has a clear impact on judgement and ability to make rational decisions.

During one session in which the Health and Community Care Committee of the Scottish Parliament took evidence about the new Scottish Mental Health Bill the point of not knowing what might happen was raised by Professor David Owens:

> There is an assumption of predictability about episodes of psychiatric illness, but that assumption is not well founded... In the long term, episodes of illness can have very unpredictable outcomes. One of my patients had a bipolar illness that was for ten years absolutely predictable by the calendar. He had six weeks up and eight weeks down, with a very rapid switch between the two. On 1 November, the patient went into a down, as predicted, but he remained there until 7 July – for no reason. He came up only because we had to give him ECT. He was deteriorating rapidly and it was a health-threatening situation. Neither he nor I could have predicated that. The assumption that there is an element of pre-dictability in both symptoms and circumstances is not valid (Scottish Parliament 2002, column 3301).

Generally, where specific law for psychiatric advance directives exists there is a requirement for the person to be capable before they can change or revoke their advance directive. In the USA this is often referred to as the Ulysses contract. In Scotland one of the same group of people who has witnessed the capacity of the person to make the advance statement has to act as witness to the person's capacity to withdraw it. (It does not have to be the same person.) Although a form is provided (Scottish Executive 2004) all the person has to write is: 'I hereby withdraw the advance statement made by me [write your name] on [write the date your advance statement was witnessed]' (p.10).

The person is reminded to let everyone who has a copy of the advance state-ment have a copy of their withdrawal statement. Interestingly any accompanying personal statement is not rescinded by this withdrawal and it is suggested it is reviewed at the same time as the withdrawal.

Although there is no formal requirement for an advance statement to be reviewed it is suggested that 'it is good practice to do so about every six months, and at least once a year'. This includes 'checking and updating everyone who has a copy'. This would certainly deal with the anxiety of some that an advance state-ment might be out-of-date when it comes to be used. With no formal system for recording this, however, it is not clear how anyone would know how recently the advance directive had been reviewed. Although the person could amend a note 'reviewed on...' on the document, their capacity at this time would not be witnessed. Changes, however, would require a new advance statement to be written and witnessed.

Other laws may require the same or some combination of court and psychiatrists or other clinicians to assess capacity to withdraw an advance directive, although some (e.g. Hawaii) may allow for the treating doctor alone to make the decision.

A particular problem arises where the making of an advance directive is implicit in legislation to make a general advance directive. In such cases it is not at all clear whether an incapacitous person can revoke a psychiatric advance directive as they could a general health care directive.

In the same way that some people have suggested that as part of the advance directive the person should make a statement about when it should be invoked, it has been suggested that they should also make a statement about whether they can revoke it at any time, or only when they are capable (Winick 1996).

CHAPTER 12

The Experience of Advance Directives in Clinical Practice

There is limited evidence concerning how psychiatric advance directives are 'working' in practice. The literature includes a few experiential studies, some observational or naturalistic studies and accounts of individuals' personal experiences. Although some general conclusions can be drawn in limited areas the different types of advance directives and legal restrictions, styles of introducing and using them, and setting of mental health services make generalisations a risky endeavour. To this end the studies tend to be reported independently so that the differences are not lost.

The main areas with some evidence of how advance directives are being experienced are:

- uptake of advance directives

- invoking advance directives

- contents of advance directives

- outcome measures.

Attitudes to the use of advance directives will be considered in the next chapter. Little has been written about the process of introducing the idea of advance directives to service providers, or in any detail to service users. This may reflect the nature of the research process and articles which focus on research methodology and results. Thomas (2003) makes passing reference to this. The only major study describing the process of introducing advance agreements as policy and liaising with service providers and users is that of Wauchope (2006).

Uptake of advance directives

The research carried out so far suggests that, even for people with a chronic major mental illness, the uptake of advance directives may not be as high as might have been expected by supporters of advance directives unless there is specific intervention to support people making one. The various forms of advance directives may have a differential impact on uptake but there is no clear information on this. Also, it might be expected that uptake in research studies would be higher than that in standard clinical practice.

Backlar and McFarland (1996, 1998) employed a questionnaire to look at the use of advance directives in Oregon. The law there allows for patients both to stipulate their own wishes in an advance directive and to appoint an adult to act as their representative to follow their wishes should they lose capacity.

More than 4500 questionnaires were sent out with a newsletter to three organisations for families and care providers of people with 'severe and persistent mental disorders'. A further 107 questionnaires were sent to the medical directors of mental health programmes. From this large sample only 156 replies were received (23 from families and 133 from providers), reporting on 64 completed advance directives. In 40 of these, a surrogate decision-maker was identified. Where the diagnosis of the person making the advance directive was known, this was predominantly schizophrenia (47%) or affective disorder (37%).

The disappointingly low response rate seemed to be related to the number of respondents who had never heard of advance directives or their availability under Oregon law. An interesting insight was offered by one respondent, however, in a note attached to the questionnaire. A psychologist wrote: 'Because I practise in a rural area where resources are poor, I use the advance directive as an information tool and part of my treatment methodology' (Backlar and McFarland 1996, p.1389).

This suggests the possibility of targeting advance directives at patients who may be discriminated against in terms of resources, whether this is through geography (as in this case) or individual factors which make the patients disadvantaged in their local service provision area.

A later study by Backlar et al. (2001) took a convenience sample of 40 patients with 'severe and persistent mental disorders' from two sites in Oregon. Of these, 30 made a psychiatric advance directive, although it should be noted that participants were paid to take part in the research interview.

A study offering an opportunity to make an independent crisis card or agreed joint crisis card was offered to patients in Camberwell, South London (Sutherby et al. 1999). To meet the criteria patients had to have had at least two hospital admissions, one of which had to be in the previous two years, and to have an ICD diagnosis of schizophrenia, bipolar affective disorder, depressive disorder with psychotic symptoms or other psychotic disorder. Of the 106 patients who met the criteria, 40 per cent wanted to make a crisis card. Comparing demographic variables for those who wanted to make a card with those who did not, those who did were significantly more likely to be white, have an affective psychosis, to have been ill longer and to have attempted suicide or have been assessed as at risk of suicide. Using logistic regression, the three variables distinguishing the two groups were diagnosis, frequency of admission (less frequent more likely to agree) and history of suicide attempts/assessed risk of suicide.

Geller (2000) used a case note method to find out how many patients in a state hospital in Massachusetts had an advance directive in the form of a health care proxy. Of the 161 patients in the hospital only 10 per cent had a valid health care proxy. The main reason for there being no proxy was incompetency. Of the 33 per cent of patients who had a proxy in their charts, 21 per cent of patients had refused to sign them. Of the 23 per cent of patients who had no proxy 17 per cent of the total had a substituted judgement decision made by a court, so would not be able to make a valid proxy. Geller concluded that only 6 per cent of patients who could have had proxies affecting treatment did not have one.

The studies reported above looked at clinical practice. The following studies concern programmes promoting or researching advance directives.

Srebnik et al. (2003), as part of a larger study, asked patients in two counties in Washington State about their interest in making an advance directive. Patients had to be over 18 years and to have had at least two visits to the psychiatric emergency department or hospitalisations in the previous two years. Furthermore, they had to be able to take part in the research interviews in English. From electronic records 475 patients were identified, of whom 317 (67%) could be traced and 303 (64%) were eligible to take part. Those not eligible could either not consent, not speak enough English or were unwell. In total 161 (53%) patients expressed an interest in making an advance directive.

In 257 (85%) cases there was sufficient information to look at factors which might influence uptake. Using bivariate analysis the individual factors which were influential were: having a major depressive illness, not having schizophrenia and not having been hospitalised nor having an outpatient commitment order in the past two years. The other important factor was having a case manager supporting making an advance directive. These factors were then entered into a logistic regression analysis. The only variables positively associated with showing an interest in making advance directives were having no previous outpatient commitment orders and having a supportive case manager.

In a study in Bradford, England, by Thomas and Cahill (2004) they commented that 'two years of extensive development work with service users and mental health professionals generated a disappointingly low uptake of advance statements' (p.123). The low uptake comprised one person out of 70 service users.

As part of their major study on advance directives Swanson et al. (2006b) looked at the uptake of psychiatric advance directives (PADs) in five American states: California, Florida, Illinois, Massachusetts and North Carolina. These represented 'a diversity of statutory approaches'. Across the sites the mean age of the

1011 respondents was 41–47 years. Across the different states the numbers who had an advance instruction ranged from 2 to 7 per cent, and who had authorised a proxy from 2 to 5 per cent. In total the percentage who had one or both ranged from 4 to 13 per cent. The number who did not have a PAD but who said they wanted one (any type) was 66 to 77 per cent. There was greatest support for a combined PAD (68%) with only 18 per cent wanting a stand-alone advance instruction and 14 per cent wanting a power of attorney without additional instruction. Demand for PADs was greatest amongst those who were women, non-white, with a history of self-harm, arrest and decreased personal autonomy, and who felt pressure to comply with medication. Having greater insight, having benefits controlled by another and feeling external pressure to keep outpatient appointments made it more likely the person would have completed a PAD.

The importance of staff involvement in the uptake of advance directives was demonstrated by Swanson *et al.* (2006c). They looked at the use of facilitators to assist in the making of psychiatric advance directives and to overcome the major barriers to uptake. This intervention was described as: 'A semi-structured, manualised interview and guided discussion of choices involved in anticipatory mental health treatment planning…includes orientation to concepts related to psychiatric advance directives, review of past treatment experiences and documentation of future treatment preferences' (p.1944).

Also included was information on the law in North Carolina. There are three choices for an advance directive: either a stand-alone advance instruction, the appointment of a power of attorney or a combination of both. On average the intervention sessions took two hours.

The control group was given an introduction to psychiatric advance directives at the end of the baseline interview along with written material describing them, copies of standard forms and the free phone number 'of the local consumer organisation that provides consultation to persons who wish to prepare psychiatric advance directives'.

Of the 523 persons eligible 51 (10%) declined to take part in the study. Of the 469 included, 239 were assigned to the facilitated intervention group and 230 to the control group. Of the 469 asked if they wanted to complete a PAD if they were offered assistance, 89 per cent (419) said they would. Four people (1%) already had a PAD.

The characteristics of those in the study were: 60 per cent female, 58 per cent African-American, 38 per cent white, 11 per cent married/co-habiting, 28 per cent less than high school education, 57 per cent living independently, and 23 per cent had worked for pay in the last month. Forty-nine per cent had a diagnosis of schizophrenia or related psychotic disorder, 27 per cent had bipolar disorder and 14 per cent had depression with psychotic features.

Sixty-five patients (27%) refused to meet with the facilitator after randomisation (only three of whom already had an advance directive), leaving 174 patients. Of these, 146 (84% or 61% of the total) made an advance directive, with the majority, 103 (70%), completing both an advance instruction and power of attorney. Thirty-two (22% completed only the advance instruction and 11 (7%) completed only the power of attorney. No information is given over whether or not completing a power of attorney was linked to the person being unable to identify an appropriate person.

In the control group one person had a pre-existing PAD. A further seven advance directives were completed: three advance instructions, one power of attorney and three completed both.

Factors which predicted making an advance directive were age (above 44 years), reasoning ability, adverse experience with medication, and being independently motivated to seek help. The only negative predictor was a recent history of violent victimisation.

These differences are not just significantly different but dramatically so: 61 per cent of the total against 3 per cent. It is noteworthy that this is despite the control group being given what might be seen as a reasonable amount of information and guidance on making a PAD. Indeed, this is likely to be more than many services provide. It should not be surprising, however, since a substantial body of work from health promotion and behaviour change indicates that having the behaviour easily available (whether this be anything from a dental check-up to healthy food) made uptake of the new behaviour more likely.

The interest in 'joint' advance directives in the USA – those which combine advance instructions and power of attorney – may not apply in other legal jurisdictions (such as Britain) where there is not a history of appointing a person to make health care decisions (although there is for financial decisions). It would be interesting to know people's views on this in such jurisdictions.

These studies are reported separately as it is difficult to draw any clear conclusions about level of uptake. The range is wide, and in part seems to depend on how and why patients were asked. One important issue in reporting uptake is the denominator use. The impact of this shows itself if figures from some of the studies are reworked using different denominators. For example, the 53 per cent of eligible patients who said they were interested in making an advance directive reduces to 34 per cent of the total population identified through patient records (Srebnik *et al.* 2003). The requirements of a clinical trial influenced who was deemed eligible by Papageorgiou *et al.* (2002), who did not report uptake as such. It can be worked out, however, from the figures given. Here, relevant figures are not for those who actually completed the Preference for Care booklet, but those who agreed to take part in the trial (and thus were presumably willing and competent to complete the booklet). One hundred and sixty-one agreed to take part and 27 did not, giving an uptake rate of 86 per cent. The number assessed for the project, however, was 605, which reduces the uptake to 27 per cent. That 61 per cent were excluded from the study because of remaining on a section of the Mental Health Act or being transferred to another hospital is a decision of the researchers and reflects the outcomes they impose, rather than a choice of the patients. The very high uptake rate here from those eligible might reflect a group of patients coming to the end of a period of detention and compulsory treatment and may not be representative of other groups of patients.

In the Swanson *et al.* study (2006c) the original number screened for inclusion was 363 of whom 116 (18% were not included, either being deemed ineligible (no reasons given) or for other reasons (not given). A further 51 (8% of the total, 10% of those eligible) declined. If it is assumed that the total group would have been split evenly between the control and intervention groups (i.e. 318 in each group) the 146 who completed a PAD reduces further from 61 per cent to 46 per cent.

Invoking advance directives

The research trials on advance directives are less than illuminating on when they were invoked. The first statement in the Preferences of Care booklet (Papageorgiou *et al.* 2002, 2004) outlines the signs that the patient is becoming ill and what happened just before they were put on a section or became ill previously. It was not made clear if these are intended as triggers for consulting the other choices in the booklet. Since the main outcome measured was reduction in involuntary commitment, it might appear that it was when this was being considered that the 'directive' would be triggered. The time and process for using the booklet was not clear from the published reports and the low use, and even awareness of it by psychiatrists. This might suggest this was not clear to them either.

The joint crisis plan introduced by Henderson *et al.* (2004) also used reduction of compulsory admission or treatment and other admission as its outcome measures. Again, no indication of how the plans were invoked is given but the assumption is when these circumstances arise. In neither study is the use of these advance agreements overtly linked to the formal assessment of, or definition of, incapacity.

Although not describing when actually used Srebnik *et al.* (2005) reported on the decisions taken by patients in their advance directive on when they should be invoked. Almost half (47%) linked activation to the point of legal incapacity, 24 per cent linked it to hospital admission, and 22 per cent to using crisis services. Srebnik later discussed a number of capacity issues involved in both invoking and revoking advance directives (Srebnik and Kim 2006).

Contents of advance directives

The heart of an advance directive is what it contains: what it asks to happen or not happen and then whether this is delivered. It is also the area which causes professionals most consternation – in so far as how does the advance directive compromise their clinical integrity. As outlined in the previous chapter, different frameworks for writing advance directives may lead patients to make decisions in specific areas, or discount others. It is not, therefore, possible to conduct a meta-analysis of all choices, although some, such as medication, will appear in all examples of advance directives. Surprisingly, the content is not always of interest to researchers – or at least not in what they report. Henderson *et al.* (2004), for example, made no mention of the joint crisis plan choices on 'advance statements of preferences for care'.

Sherman (1998) reported limited information on the contents of advance directives using a computer program, but covered two areas of 'hotly debated' concern. In terms of naming an agent or proxy, 82 per cent (32/39) patients did so, and only two people (2/54, 4%) refused all medication. All other patients agreed to specific medications/combinations/dosages or consented to medication as proposed by the attending psychiatrist, although some (number unspecified) wanted their outpatient psychiatrist also to agree to the medication.

The few studies which look at the contents of advance directives are worth considering in some detail. Since there is no work comparing types of advance directive, contents (among other things) may depend both on who completes the advance directive and how the directive is presented. The best that can be managed is some comparison between studies (imperfect though this might be).

As well as headings of 'contact details' and 'current care and treatment plan' the joint crisis plan developed by Sutherby *et al.* (1999) had future plans under the headings 'care in crises' and 'practical help in a crisis'. Under the four headings 'care in a crisis', 90 per cent (36) completed 'What I would like done when I first become unwell'. This included making contact with their treatment team (83%). In 61 per cent of cases this included further statements about care. 'Circumstances in which I would want to be admitted to hospital for treatment' was completed by 70 per cent and 65 per cent completed preferred treatment or social care during a crisis or relapse. Finally 53 per cent gave 'specific refusals regarding treatment during a crisis or a relapse'. This was mainly refusal of specific medication (alone or in combination) because of side-effects. No one refused all drugs, or all classes of drugs (e.g. antipsychotics).

Practical help in a crisis was fairly limited. A person to be contacted on admission to hospital with specific requests, such as 'Check my home is secure' was requested by 53 per cent and only two patients (5%) made arrangements for children or dependants. A catchall heading of 'Other information I would like to be known or taken into account (e.g. special diet, people to be told/not told, etc.)' was only completed by 20 per cent. Those selected by patients as who they wanted to have a copy of the crisis card were: themself and their treatment team, 100 per cent; the emergency clinic, 85 per cent; their nominee, 75 per cent; their general practitioner, 73 per cent; and other, 53 per cent.

A study of attitudes to advance directives in Oregon resulted in 30 patients making one (Backlar *et al.* 2001). No one refused all treatment, although some treatments were refused and 27 per cent specifically refused haloperidol and 57 per cent electro-convulsive therapy (ECT). Twenty per cent wanted to continue on their current treatment and 20 per cent chose to accept their doctor's treatment decisions. Other, non-treatment issues include 'privacy when I go to the bathroom' and 'I'd rather go to (named) hospital than jail'.

In a small, qualitative study with ten people who had made an advance directive Amering *et al.* (2005) also found that no one refused all treatment. Nor did anyone 'seize upon it to make a point or lodge a grievance'. The study was not primarily focused on the content of the directive, but some examples were given. These included: 'favoured coping strategies (such as being left alone at times or listening to music) and 'boundary rules' (such as not being touched by staff without being asked). Treatment choices (medications and dosages) and refusals (such as ECT) were also outlined, along with reasons for the choices. People they wanted to see along with those they did not were also listed. The researchers reported that there was concern that the advance directives were 'feasible'.

Papageorgiou *et al.* (2004) gave a detailed breakdown of the responses in their Preferences of Care booklet. They reported that patients gave 'logical and consistent answers' in response to what they would like if they became ill again. Eighty patients were able to make up to three choices. Although a total of 240 choices were thus possible only 155 were made. There is no comment on whether most people only made two choices or whether approximately one-third only made one choice. No examples are given of the patients' choices, nor is there an explanation given for how categories were derived from these responses. It is not clear, therefore, what the patient was asking for (for example the heading 'more service input'). No category reached even one-third of patients wanting that option. The top two with 29 per cent were 'more talking therapies' and 'more service input'. This was followed by 'support to take medication' 25 per cent, 'family and/or social support' 23 per cent, 'see my GP' 22 per cent, 'more and better communication with professionals' 18 per cent, 'treatment in the community' 13 per cent, 'better housing/financial conditions' 6 per cent and 'to see a lawyer' 4 per cent.

Two separate questions asked what the patient would want or not want if they had to be admitted to hospital. Only 73 responses are recorded for what patients would not want, suggesting that at least seven patients did not complete this section at all, although the number could be higher if multiple responses were made by some patients. The main category of response was 'force/coercion/intrusion', recorded by 43 per cent. The next largest category was 'admission by unknown staff' 16 per cent, and 'particular treatment' 15 per cent (although what these were was not specified in the article). The next largest category was 'human rights not respected' 8 per cent, 'others informed 6 per cent and 'unwanted contact from family' 4 per cent.

What was wanted gave rise to 103 responses. The largest category was 'better quality hospital facilities' 43 per cent, followed by 'treatments/therapies (e.g. alternative therapies, counselling, psychotherapy)' 33 per cent; 'improved human rights' 32 per cent; 'more say/explanations in treatment' 14 per cent, and 'avoidance of coercion' 9 per cent.

There were 72 responses to the question about who to contact, including one person who stated no one. If it is assumed that the five people who did not want anyone informed and the three who did not want 'unwanted contact from family' make up the missing eight patients, eleven per cent of patients did not want family informed of their admission. This contrasts with the 52 per cent of patients who wanted their family contacted, 13 per cent who wanted 'other services' (rehabilitation hostels, social worker, CPN) informed, 11 per cent who wanted friends contacted and 6 per cent who wanted their GP, 5 per cent their consultant and 3 per cent their lawyer told.

These results are interesting in a number of ways. Nothing is said specifically about refusing medication but even if all 12 who were refusing treatment were refusing medication this is still less than the 20 who want support to take it. The emphasis on avoidance of force and coercion might be expected from a group of patients who were coming to the end of a period of commitment under the Mental Health Act. What is not clear from the description given is whether the patients were asking for earlier intervention to avoid commitment or whether they were wanting to be left alone. If the latter, there is no indication of whether the likelihood of this happening was discussed with the patients. This, tied to the 32 per cent who wanted improved human rights (not specified as to what this meant), would benefit from further elaboration.

Another response where compliance might be difficult is the 13 patients who did not want to be admitted by unknown staff. Staff turnover, staff absence and an emergency situation may all contribute to making this problematic. If all the responses to what people do not want are taken together then 73 per cent fall into this category. This would seem to be setting up the advance directives to fail. If this is coupled with the 43 per cent of responses which want 'better quality hospital facilities', the purpose of the Preferences of Care booklet starts to look uncertain. Although it is more than reasonable that patients want good quality hospital facilities, whether an advance directive is the most appropriate way of achieving this is open to question. That 14 per cent of patients stated they wanted 'more say' if they had 'to be admitted to hospital again' also suggests that maybe they did not see the choices they were making in the booklet as contributing much to this future treatment.

Another study which looked in some detail at the contents of advance directives was that of Srebnik *et al.* (2005), involving 106 patients in Washington State, who used the computer programme AD-Maker. Of these 81 per cent listed at least one preferred medication and 64 per cent at least one they wanted to refuse. Again no one refused all medication. First generation antipsychotics were the most refused (35%), followed by antidepressants and mood stabilisers (15% each). The two groups most preferred were antidepressants (54%) and second generation antipsychotics (53%).

The reasons given for refusing different medications given in 64 per cent of the advance directives from a specified list were: side-effects 45 per cent; 'feeling "doped up and foggy"' 32 per cent; the 'medications "don't help"' 29 per cent; the person could not engage in 'normal everyday activities' 28 per cent; the medication made 'mental problems worse' 15 per cent; they were allergic to medication 15 per cent, and 14 per cent gave other reasons. These included 'increased blood pressure, weight gain, kidney problems, sexual dysfunction, muscle rigidity, gait problems and oedema'.

All but two people responded to a list of options about whether they would try medications not listed in the advance directives. The responses were: 'if side-effects could be eliminated' 36 per cent; 'if prescribed by an outpatient physician' 30 per cent; 'if prescribed by an inpatient physician' 19 per cent, and 13 per cent were unwilling to take any medication not listed in the directive.

The majority (68%) of patients preferred an alternative to hospital admission, although 25 per cent preferred hospitalisation. Although some of the alternatives chosen (from a specified list) indicated where the person would stay, not all did. Those that indicated overnight support were: 'stay overnight at a crisis or respite bed' 42 per cent; 'stay overnight with a friend' or 'with family' 16 per cent for each; have a friend or family member stay with them, 9 per cent and 5 per cent respectively; and one person wanted to stay in a woman's shelter. Of the alternatives which did not mention accommodation were 'see prescriber to help with medications' 47 per cent; 'have someone I could call' 42 per cent; have someone call them 38 per cent; and one person wanted to use marijuana.

A third of advance directives gave no instructions on this point. Despite this 80 per cent listed a preferred hospital and 48 per cent specified hospitals to avoid with only 20 per cent not giving any instructions. It would seem, therefore, that even though they might not want to be admitted to hospital, about half accepted that it was a possibility. The most frequently listed hospital to avoid was the state hospital. The most frequent reason given (from a specified list) for wanting to avoid a particular hospital was 'poor quality care' 29 per cent, followed by 'staff not treating clients with respect' 21 per cent, 'problems with patients being hurt or abused' 16 per cent, and that it was at an 'inconvenient location for family and friends to visit' 8 per cent. Other reasons given included 'having treatment provided involuntarily at the facility', the facility 'having too many rules' which included no smoking, and 'not having enough safety or support'.

Almost three-quarters of patients (72%) wanted to refuse ECT whilst 16 per cent would consent to ECT. Of these, three gave specific instructions regarding voltage and maximum number of treatments (one or two). There is no indication of whether the patients had any experience of ECT or whether it was likely to be a treatment possibility and had been discussed. This decision could be based on hearsay and stigma rather than experience. This is in contrast to the medication decisions where patients chose which medications to list and thus these were more likely to be based on experience.

An interesting and important set of choices offered in AD-Maker (Srebnik *et al.* 2005), and not usually elsewhere, is what the person wants to happen in an emergency. Lists of specified choices were offered in two forms: de-escalation methods and seclusion, restraint and sedation. Eighty-nine per cent of advance directives listed options under both of these. Of the de-escalation methods 'time out or privacy' was the most common choice 38 per cent; followed by 'talk me down' 14 per cent, and 'help me vent or examine my feelings' 10 per cent. Other options were 'decrease stimulation around me' 8 per cent; 'offer me more medications' 8 per cent; and 'divert my attention to something else' 5 per cent. One person opted for 'have neutral person settle the dispute' and one person opted for each of the 'other' instructions of 'calling a specific person, music or art, sleep, hot tea or going for a walk'. Of the options listed the rank order of choices was: 'medication in pill form' 42 per cent; 'seclusion alone' 24 per cent; 'medication via injection' 14 per cent; 'medication in liquid form' 7 per cent; and 'seclusion plus restraint' 2 per cent.

The treatment preferences were rated for their clinical utility by at least one psychiatrist. At least 95 per cent of the directives were rated as 'feasible, useful, and consistent with practice standards'. The only exception was instructions about willingness to accept medication not listed in the advance directive due to a small number of patients who were not prepared to accept such medication 'under any circumstances'.

AD-Maker also allows for non-treatment decisions to be made. These were reported in less detail. Eighty-one per cent named people to be notified of admission to hospital. These were, in rank order: parents, siblings, friends, clinicians, spouses and children. A minority (27%) gave details of people they did not want to visit if they were hospitalised. These were, in the main, first-degree relatives, friends or spouses.

Half (48%) of the directives named someone to manage finances whilst the patient was in hospital. These were, in order: case manager, parents, siblings, friends and spouses. A minority named people to care for pets (14%) or dependants (6%). Nearly half (46%) appointed a surrogate decision-maker. These were in order: a friend, parents, sibling, spouse or child.

From a list of dietary preferences 42 per cent of directives had choices about diet. This listed foods to be avoided, mainly sugar, salt, meats, acidic foods and fats. No mention was made of specific religious dietary requirements (e.g. kosher, halal).

A list of 'assistive devices' was provided from which 59 per cent selected at least one to be retained whilst they were in hospital. These were almost all 'corrective lenses' or dentures/plates.

Lastly, in the 'other' category 30 per cent of directives had additional instructions. These were usually treatment for medical conditions, 'wanting to have someone to talk to during a crisis. To be able to sleep, or to do art or other expressive activities'. Again, at least 95 per cent 'were rated as feasible, useful, and consistent with practice standards'.

These studies may help to lay to rest some of the concerns held by some clinicians who fear for large numbers of patients refusing all treatment and filling hospital wards. It may be that providing lists of choices and requiring people to complete particular sections leads to 'more realistic' choices or, as Srebnik and colleagues (2005) phrase it 'optimised the documents' clinical utility' but there is no real evidence for this.

In all the studies people currently engaged with services were involved, and in the Washington study 'may have been more likely than others (patients) to provide instructions in advance directives consistent with familiar usual care' (Srebnik et al. 2005). The choices in the London study (Papageorgiou et al. 2004), which have a different focus, may reflect the concerns of patients who had recently been detained as much as a different form of completing the advance directive. Where agreements have been made with staff still other considerations may apply (Henderson et al. 2004; Sutherby et al. 1999).

In the study by Swanson et al. (2006c) of 136 advance instructions, again reassuringly for worried clinicians, no one refused all medication. Although 77 per cent refused one or more psychotropic medications, 93 per cent gave advance consent to one or more psychotropic medications. This is further evidence that patients have clear views on what helps them or otherwise. Refusal of ECT treatment was endorsed by 58 per cent. Eighty-nine per cent gave advance consent to admission to one or more named hospitals and 62 per cent refused admission to one or more named hospitals.

Of other instructions; 98.5 per cent gave contacts for a crisis (65% therapist, 55% psychiatrists, 42% primary care physician); 76.5 per cent wanted to be treated with respect; 57 per cent wanted to avert the use of seclusion and restraints; and 39 per cent had other medical information or instructions.

Of the proxies identified (105), one-third were a sibling or parent (34% each); 19 per cent were offspring; 17 per cent a friend; and 7 per cent a spouse or significant other. Almost all were granted full authority: consent to psychotropic medication (99%); consent to hospitalisation (97%); hire and fire health care providers (97%); and review medical records (94%).

The advance directives were rated blindly by psychiatrists as to their 'consistency with community practice standards in North Carolina'. There was an overall 90.5 per cent endorsement of them being 'consistent, feasible and useful'. The clinical information was rated as useful in 94 per cent, the medication preferences as consistent and feasible in 90.5 per cent and the hospital preferences as consistent and feasible in 83 per cent.

Some individual examples of advance directives are given in the literature. A brief description (anonymous 2004) of what is called 'notes on care' gives, along with standard information about contact details and who is to be informed, details about how to keep the person safe. These include taking away car keys, with a reminder that a spare set might be in her handbag and that there may be accumulated drugs in the car. The patient reports a very positive response to this from her care team. A very wide advance directive is described by Dace (2001), specifying how she would like to be treated in hospital as well as medication refusal, which received different responses by different clinicians.

Outcome measures

As already mentioned there is no agreed outcome for advance directives and different studies have used different measures. It is not possible, therefore, to draw any clear conclusions about their impact. Even where similar measures are used, the different timing of the introduction of the directive and the different styles of directive make comparisons problematic and conclusions uncertain.

The joint crisis cards developed by Sutherby et al. (1999) were completed by 40 patients, of whom 26 had a crisis during the follow-up period. In 73 per cent of these cases the crisis card was consulted. Sixty-one per cent were admitted to hospital at least once, and for 81 per cent the card was consulted. There was a 30 per cent reduction in admission during the follow-up period.

In 74 per cent of those consulted the card was deemed useful by either the patient or the key worker, although this reduced to about half (54%) if the total number of cards available is considered. Areas where the card was deemed particularly useful were providing information on carers and current treatment where the patient was involved with the police (12%) or was unwell or treated outside their local area (23%). They also helped in the assessment of the crisis in recognising triggers and early signs of relapse. Admissions were reduced in this group (compared to figures for the previous two years) and it was thought they either averted unnecessary admissions or, in some cases, facilitated early admission. Ten nominees were contacted and attended.

In terms of treatment plans, 9 of the 21 who had refused specific treatment were admitted to hospital and in all but one case 'the requests were met without difficulty'. In one case a man was given haloperidol against his wishes, despite staff consulting his care plan, 'because of the seriousness of the emergency' although the authors report that 'it would have been feasible to carry out the instructions'. They attributed this, and another incident involving a hospital admission, as occurring 'early in the study period' when it seemed that 'acceptance of the validity of the instructions was only partial.'

Two studies in London carried out within a couple of years of each other came to opposite conclusions about outcomes. Papageorgiou *et al.* (2004) used the previously described Preferences for Care booklet with 79 patients. The main outcome measure was 'the rate of compulsory re-admissions' with a secondary outcome of time spent in hospital either voluntarily or compulsorily in the 12 months following discharge. There was no significant difference between the groups with an advance directive and the control group without. In the former, 19 per cent of patients were re-admitted and in the latter 21 per cent. Nor was there any difference in the number of compulsory or voluntary admissions, nor days spent in hospital. The Self-Efficacy Scale was used to assess patients' 'ability to make decisions and conduct their lives' with no significant difference between groups.

The authors presented several reasons for the lack of impact, but dismissed most of them. Arguing that patients near discharge, although assessed as competent, may 'not have had the capacity to make full use of the directives', including problems with insight and concentration, was set against the argument that patients were assessed by experienced clinicians. In follow-up, however, one patient suggested the reason why their advance directive was not used was because they were not thinking clearly when it was written (Papageorgiou *et al.* 2004). It was also suggested that the statistical power may have been compromised by fewer than expected compulsory admissions, but the difference in the two groups is so small as to make this unlikely.

Lack of resources, changes in key workers and the directive being 'regarded as an administrative burden by staff, who assumed their management already took account of patients' wishes' may have contributed to their lack of use. The authors suggested that these 'are not uncommon features of psychiatric services in large metropolitan areas, and are an expected part of any naturalistic setting'. That the advance directive was drawn up with 'someone independent of the patient's care' might have diminished 'the treating professionals' sense of "ownership" or commitment to honour the terms of the directive'. Although this may well be true and have contributed to the low use, it is, nevertheless, a somewhat strange position. The point of advance directives, surely, is that they are owned by patients and not staff. This may have reflected a view that such directives should more properly be agreements.

An indication of this is given in the last suggestion by the authors that the directives might not have been practical but dismissed this as, during drafting, 'any directive considered to be impractical was amended after discussion with staff'. This was to deal with appropriate requests which, nevertheless, might not be able to be met, such as admission to a single room.

The main reason for no difference, however, may be more fundamental (Atkinson *et al.* 2005; Geller 2003). Despite referring to the booklet as an advance directive it was not really this, but a statement of preferences and, in many ways, closer to an advance agreement. Although the main outcome measure was compulsory hospitalisation the preferences stated were 'not intended to address compulsory admissions directly', which seems inconsistent. Since, in addition, it was stated that staff did not have to comply with the choices made it is difficult to see what the Preferences for Care booklet would achieve, or why the patient should expect it to make a difference.

Although there was no description of the standards of treatment the control group experienced, or their relationship with their psychiatrist and treating team, it is easy to believe that many of the preferences expressed by the intervention group may also have been expressed by the control group and that, in reality, there was very little difference in either the process or what happened to the two groups.

Thomas (2003) questioned the power balance in both the directive and the study. This goes beyond the straightforward acknowledgement that stated preferences could be over-ridden. He asked questions about who carried out recruitment, and how, about the amount of information patients were given about advance directives, including pros and cons, and how both staff and patients were involved in discussions about how the advance directive fitted in with current structures of service delivery, such as the Care Programme Approach.

The researchers replied with full answers to these questions (King, Papageorgiou and Dawson 2003), indicating that, as far as possible, full and even 'extensive' discussions were held with stakeholders. They did, however, acknowledge 'obtaining funding for this valuable work is extremely difficult, and it was thus limited' and went on to assert 'ours was a pragmatic trial in which we sought to assess whether such directives were useful in a real, inner-city clinical setting'. How far this was achieved can be assessed by looking at the numbers lost to follow-up. There were no differences between the two groups in the numbers lost to follow-up, being 25 per cent in the intervention group and 29 per cent in the control group, nor in the reasons for this loss.

Even bearing in mind the 'legal complexities' which led to 'a clause stating that users' wishes could be over-ridden' it seems unlikely that this methodology could clearly answer their aim, 'to test one bold claim...namely that they (advance directives) may reduce the need for patients to be civilly committed at a later time'. To test this would really require a focus on opt-in directives and (more than likely) a range of alternatives to hospital that patients are willing to accept at an early stage in their relapse or crisis. It may also raise questions about how incapacitated a person must be before the advance directive is activated.

Henderson *et al.* (2004) also used the same outcomes, reversing them so use of the Mental Health Act was a secondary outcome and admission to hospital and length of time in hospital were the primary measures in their version of advance agreements (joint crisis plans).

On the primary outcome of hospital admission a smaller proportion of numbers was admitted from the intervention group (30%) than in the control group (44%) but this did not reach significance. There was no difference between the two groups in the mean number of days they spent in hospital although clearly there were wide individual differences. In total about a quarter of patients had an admission lasting more than one month (23% in the intervention group and 29% in the control group).

For the secondary outcome measure, however – compulsory admission and treatment – there was a significant difference. In the intervention group 13 per cent had at least one compulsory admission, compared with 27 per cent (20/80) in the control group. The length of time on section was similar for the two groups: a mean of 114 days (median 104) for the intervention group and 117 (median 99) for the control group.

An economic evaluation was also carried out (Flood *et al.* 2006). In use of services, as well as fewer psychiatric admissions, patients in the joint crisis plan groups (compared to the control group) also had fewer attendances at outpatient clinics, accident and emergency services and day centres, and fewer contacts with social workers and criminal justice staff. They had more non-psychiatric hospital admissions, more contact with general practitioners and community psychiatric nurses and more use of specialised accommodation.

Over 15 months the mean total cost for patients in the joint crisis plan group was £37,264 (US$13,560, €10,616) and for the control group £8,359 (US$15,609, €12,217). Although lower, this difference was not significant. The actual difference of £1,095 would need to be increased to £3,381 for the difference to be significant, which represents a further 14 days in hospital per patient. Despite the difference not being significant, any saving of money might be welcomed by hard-pressed managers if there were no lowering of other outcomes.

Using a cost-effectiveness acceptability curve, Flood *et al.* concluded 'that there is at least a 78 per cent probability that the joint crisis plan is more cost-effective than standardised service information in preventing admissions'.

No information is given on the content of the joint crisis plan to achieve either fewer days in hospital or less use of the Mental Health Act. Given less use of other services, greater compliance with medication might be suspected, but this is not confirmed.

Henderson *et al.* (2004) pointed out that 'the provision of a written care plan, signed by the patient, is now required in England'. They contrasted this with a joint crisis plan (which seems to be used synonymously), which is voluntary. Whether the distinction was clear to patients is uncertain. It also raises the question of whether, if only a minority of patients take it up, this really matters if the main outcome is for the patient's wishes to be adhered to. If, however, the main outcomes are seen as use of services (for example admission days) or service delivery (for example through the Mental Health Act) then this is a different matter.

CHAPTER 13

Attitudes to Advance Directives

Advance directives will only 'take off', gain currency and make an impact on patients' care and lives if all those involved see them as worthwhile and useful. This means that patients have to want to make them as much as professionals have to agree to implement them. From this perspective both sets of views are equally important, and likely to influence each other. If patients see no point in advance directives they will never develop in a meaningful way. If, however, professionals are negative about them (or at least not enthusiastic) then why should patients see them as important (at least where they have no legal currency)? The previous chapter indicated that patients were more likely to complete an advance directive if they were assisted or supported by staff. This would suggest that educating and motivating staff is at least as important as educating and encouraging patients. So far little account had been taken of families and their role in, and attitudes to, advance directives.

A number of studies examine both mental health professionals' and patients' views. These are either in the abstract (where respondents have no experience of advance directives), at the initial stage with a view to making them, or after some experience of using them. The paucity of studies actually using advance directives and looking at outcomes means that there is very little evidence of the latter. Attitudes to specific dimensions have already been covered in Chapter 4.

Patients' attitudes to advance directives

Backlar *et al.* (2001) reported patients' views on the process of making an advance directive, although the directive itself had not yet been used. Of a group of 30 patients, 87 per cent approved of them. The majority of responses indicated that the patients felt empowered, for example: 'I have a strong desire of protection if I get hospitalised. I know what they'll be giving me, I hope'.

Papageorgiou and colleagues (2004) followed up 59 (75% of total) patients in the Preferences for Care arm of their trial one year after discharge from hospital. Although a majority (75%) remembered drawing up the document only about half (48%) said they still had it and a quarter (28%) could show it to the interviewer. The responses to other questions seemed somewhat inconsistent. Fifteen patients had been re-admitted in the time frame but only two patients reported it being used in the past year with 37 per cent not knowing. Despite this, 15 per cent reported that it was useful. The reasons given, however, may help to explain this apparent discrepancy as many had little to do with treatment preferences. Instead, the reported responses were: 'helped other people understand that the patient is ill' (3); 'helped the patient to know when ill and needing admission' (2); 'helped the patient evaluate their illness' (2); 'reminded patient of things they can do to improve life' (2); and 'helped with reality testing' (1).

Although the Preferences for Care booklet might be a useful therapeutic tool it is interesting that it is acting on the patient and their responsiveness to, and responsibility for, their illness rather than acting to ensure the treatment they received from others was in accordance with their wishes. This may reflect the nature of the choices the patients were allowed to make in completing the booklet.

The reasons why it was not helpful were: staff not being aware of it or using it (17%); 'instructions not acted upon' (3%), and one each for 'written when patient not thinking clearly'; 'forgot about it'; design too bulky'; 'lost it, became out-of-date'. A number of patients (12%) indicated it had not been needed. Nevertheless, 41 per cent said they would want to use it again and 44 per cent would recommend it to others. Suggestions of how it might be improved ranged from giving it more authority, making staff more aware of it and making it more prominent in medical notes, and involving professionals more in its preparation. One suggestion – giving patients more time to complete it – possibly echoes other studies which suggest it takes patients some time to commit to making one. A practical suggestion – changing the design to make it more like a bus pass and therefore easier to carry around – echoed the design of the card produced in Oregon (Backlar 1994).

Overall, from Papageorgiou *et al.*'s study (2004) it would seem that the majority of patients either did not find the directives useful or were indifferent to them. This might reflect patients not being particularly engaged with the advance directives as presented, advance directives in general, how and when they were recruited or maybe a response to the general disinterest of the staff.

The Bazelon Centre for Mental Health Law (undated) carried out a three-year study exploring aspects of psychiatric advance directives (PADs) and collecting the views of professionals and consumers. An illuminating part of this was a qualitative reporting of consumer views. These ranged from positive to negative, there was but an acknowledgement that they could improve communication. Creating an advance directive could be empowering: 'It was very thought provoking... I found it empowering; you could stand up for yourself'. The difficulties in creating an advance directive were also acknowledged: 'It is a hard thing to do because it does bring up trauma; it does bring up past events. And it is hard, for me it was a hard thing to do. I'm glad it is over.'

As part of their major study, the team at Duke University looked at patients' preferences for PADs (Swartz *et al.* 2006). Of 456 patients, 74 per cent were interested in making a PAD involving any type of health care power of attorney and only 14 per cent wanted an advance instruction only type PAD. A further 11 per cent were not interested in either. For the groups as a whole the greatest interest was in stating treatment preferences. It was only in the latter two groups that the patients most keen to avoid unwanted treatment were interested. The greatest barriers to not completing PADs were not understanding enough (56%) and not knowing what to put in the PAD (53%). Given the possibility of appointing a proxy, 20 per cent said they did not have anyone they trusted enough to make decisions for them.

Attitudes of staff to advance directives

General views
Advance directives need staff to be positive about them if they are to be used by patients and are useful for them. Sutherby *et al.* (1999) reported that 90 per cent of key workers would recommend the crisis card they adopted to other services, but no other comments.

This is not always the case. Reporting on the process of making an advance directive, rather than their subsequent use, Backlar *et al.* (2001) indicated that although service providers were satisfied in 93 per cent of cases with the manner in which the advance directive was made with patients, 80 per cent of them nevertheless had 'serious concerns' about implementation in general. This was mainly because of a lack of institutional systems to access or implement the directive.

Atkinson *et al.* (2003b, 2004) developed five models of mental health advance directives to stimulate discussion and canvass opinion during the review of the mental health legislation in Britain. In previous discussions (Atkinson 2003b), so much emphasis had been on electro-convulsive therapy (ECT) that one model was restricted to this. It did not, however, bring up any issues not covered in other models. Two models – one patient initiated and one closer to an advance agreement – were deemed possible in the current legal context.

Using these models a postal survey was conducted of 1520 stakeholders in Britain. In total 473 (31%) responses were returned (Atkinson 2004). The response rate from Scotland was somewhat higher than from England (e.g. Directors of Social Work (SW) in Scotland, 50%, Directors of Social Services (SS) in England, 41%; psychiatrist in Scotland, 41% and in England, 25%). This may have reflected researchers based in Scotland or possibly more emphasis on advance directives in the review process.

In response to the question, 'Do you think we need advance directives?', the response from various stakeholders was: voluntary organisations, 89 per cent; Director SW/SS, 82 per cent; psychiatric nurses, 79 per cent; National Health Service (NHS) Trusts, 71 per cent; mental health officers, 66 per cent; and psychiatrists, 28 per cent. Interestingly, psychiatrists in Scotland were significantly less likely to think advance directives were needed than those in England (24% vs. 44%, $p=0.003$) although there was no explanation for this.

An analysis of themes from comments made about models suggested that even where a model was negatively viewed people still saw positive aspects in it, and across and within models many people's views were not consistent. The most positive theme was that of autonomy and empowerment with respondents positive about giving people choice and becoming involved. A hope was also expressed that the very process of making an advance directive, with the assumption that this would be made with a professional, would reduce the need for emergency treatment by encouraging early treatment. Having said that, psychiatrists were significantly less likely ($p=0.001$) than other groups to want advance directives which allowed people to opt out of treatment. Interestingly, and particularly in light of the nature of advance statements in the new Scottish legislation, in no group did a majority want to work with an opt-in advance directive. Other positive themes included seeing advance directives as encouraging responsibility, being destigmatising and a reflection of good practice. Negative themes focused on practicalities ranging from how they would be known to be valid to how they would be located.

A number of themes have positive and negative aspects, which tended to cross stakeholder groups. These included restricting clinical judgement, speed of access to treatment, childcare and finances, relationships between service users and professionals, the involvement of relatives, involvement with the law and resources. The latter point was echoed in comments about the purpose of advance directives with concern about developing a two-tier system.

A study of the views of mental health professionals in North Carolina about advance directives is presented in a series of papers (Elbogen *et al.* 2006; Swanson *et al.* 2003; Swartz *et al.* 2005; Van Dorn *et al.* 2006). Since the law there allows for advance instructions (written by the person) separately or in conjunction with the appointment of a health care power of attorney (HCPA) (or proxy) these two aspects were studied separately. Questions were asked about approval for both aspects of the state's law. A short vignette was also used, and statements about what influenced the mental health professionals' decision. There was also a 'knowledge' question regarding how the law in North Carolina defines incapacity and questions about perceptions of service system and clinical barriers to mental health care.

The response to a postal questionnaire was 32 per cent (167/578) for psychiatrists and 48 per cent (237/495) for psychologists. In addition, an online survey of clinical social workers produced 193 responses (no denominator given) (Elbogen *et al.* 2006). Amongst the psychiatrists the respondents were older (mean age 52 years, range 33–78), 71 per cent male, 87 per cent white and 43 per cent worked in the public sector setting more than 20 per cent of the time (Swartz *et al.* 2005). For the three groups taken together, however, 57 per cent of respondents were female (Elbogen *et al.* 2006).

Approval for the law on advance directives came from 54 per cent psychiatrists, 50 per cent psychologists and 38 per cent social workers. Approval for the appointment of a HCPA was slightly greater: 67 per cent of psychiatrists, 61 per cent of psychologists and 42 per cent of social workers ($p=<0.001$) (Elbogen *et al.* 2006). More psychiatrists (56%) were concerned that the benefits of advance directives could be outweighed by patients refusing medication than psychologists (42%) or social workers (39%) but these differences were not significant.

For the psychiatrists, three statistical models were carried out for both advance instructions and HCPA (Swartz *et al.* 2005). Only 38 per cent correctly answered the question about incapacity, but these psychiatrists were more likely to support advance instructions and HCPA. Generally, the more barriers within services the psychiatrists identified, the less likely they were to support either measure, possibly reflecting a view of the system's inability to implement them. Less concern about malpractice liability was associated with greater support of advance instructions, as was the importance of personal ethical practice. In contrast, more time spent in patient visits, more weight on the family's views about treatment, and importance given to the patient's suicide history were related to support of HCPA.

Across the three groups (Elbogen *et al.* 2006) there were some differences in what affected the mental health professionals' decisions to follow a patient's advance directive. Overall psychiatrists placed a greater emphasis on family opinions, therapeutic alliance and the patient's insight into their condition than the psychologists and social workers. The latter two groups put more emphasis on respecting the patient's autonomy. The authors, however, indicated that these differences should not be overestimated. All groups endorsed the importance of all these issues, and knowledge of the law was as important as these issues in deciding whether to follow an advance directive or not.

Both studies concluded that education or guidance for clinicians on the law and navigating the barriers to implementing them might result in more support for their use.

It is worth noting the lower endorsement of advance directives by social workers in the North Carolina study compared with the British study (Atkinson *et al.* 2004). This may be due to the British study anticipating the introduction of advance directives compared to the American study requiring respondents to endorse a specific law. Whether social workers in Scotland remain so positive to the newly introduced advance statements is unknown.

In the Bazelon Centre for Mental Health Law study (undated) there were, as might be expected, mixed views from providers, with concern about treatment refusal but support for opt-in directives, concern about knowing when someone had an advance directive, and how they related to civil commitment proceedings and emergency situations. Nevertheless, a number of providers indicated that PADs were a useful part of a therapeutic strategy in making 'their clinical efforts more meaningful and effective' and these were the group who were more positive about PADs.

PAD is not necessarily adversarial, but could be helpful. An example of someone for whom a PAD may be helpful is a consumer who does not talk when at a low point of mental health, but who could make a plan in advance when he/she has judgement and willingness to express it.

It was thought that there was a 'need to leave a little "wiggle room" for physicians', but most responses confirmed that more information and training were required. Generally providers preferred the appointment of a proxy to an advance instruction document, but even then urged caution over possible conflicts of interest between the consumer and the proxy. Other concerns were whether they should help consumers make advance directives. Although some thought it might bring an element of realistic expectation to the consumer, others were concerned about their possible conflict of interest.

Experience of advance directives

At one year follow-up from the patient's discharge, Papageorgiou *et al.* (2004) asked the patient's consultant for their views on the Preferences for Care booklet. Taken at face value these are fairly discouraging, but it is not always clear what it is the comments reflect. The intended outcome of the booklet was to prevent/influence compulsory admission, but specific views about that are not given. Only 15 of the 79 patients (19%) in the intervention group were re-admitted in the follow-up period, and it would have been helpful to have comments related specifically to admission and compulsory treatment. The actual number of psychiatrists who responded was not given, but responses were received for 31 patients (39%). Whether this includes all 15 who were admitted was not indicated. It may also be reasonable to assume that where there was no response the booklet had not been used or found useful.

There was no indication whether the comments on using the advance directive related to admission, preventing admission or some other outcome. Although it was reported used in only three cases (10% of responses but 4% of total group), in five cases (16% of responses, 6% of total) it was reported as 'useful in the management of the patient'. In only one of the reasons given was there a reference to capacity. In many cases the reason reflected better understanding of the patient. In one case it had been used as the 'basis of Care Programme Approach (CPA)' and in the last the response 'consultant routinely asks people about their early warning signs of stress' could as easily be counted as negative, if it is seen as adding nothing new.

What was more telling is that in only nine cases (29% of responses, 11% of total) did the psychiatrist remember its existence, and in only eight (26% of responses, 10% of total) had it been seen. This was despite a copy being sent to them, another copy being placed in the front of the patient's case notes and a briefing 'about the directives'.

Thirty-six reasons were given in the 26 responses which said the Preferences for Care booklet was not useful. The main reason was that the 'consultant/team were not aware of it' (14). In five cases it was considered that 'unrealistic preferences were given', which the authors dispute as 'something that does not fit with our data'. It might, however, indicate a difference in perspective about what is, or is not, possible or reasonable. Others claimed that it was 'not integrated into the CPA' (5). The comment that 'consultant prefers to talk face-to-face with the patient' (3) may reflect the fact that the preferences booklet was drawn up with an independent professional, which might also be the thinking behind 'not discussed with patient' (4). The former comment does, however, miss the point that it is designed to be used when the patient is unable to make a capacitous decision which is not the same as not talking to the patient. An interesting comment was that in two cases the patient did not want to use it, but the reasons for this were not given.

Although ten consultants reported it as moderately or very useful only six reported wanting to use it again. The main way in which it was believed it could be improved was to integrate it into the CPA system.

The overall sense is of a group of psychiatrists who were not interested in this, at least in part because they had not been included in the process. Although one suggested having it in an electronic format it is not clear how this would help. Since something at the front of case notes was routinely overlooked it might be overoptimistic to assume that because it is on a computer it will be read.

CHAPTER 14

Other Approaches to
Individual Future Planning

Although advance directives are generally taken as being an independent expression of future wishes, in many cases, as has been described, they are advance agreements drawn up with a member of the mental health team. In some cases there seems to be some confusion between these and joint crisis plans, which should possibly be treated differently.

Another feature of advance directives in some jurisdictions is the power to appoint a proxy or surrogate decision-maker, or durable or enduring power of attorney (DPA/DPOA or EPA). Since not all legislation allows for this, and appointing someone to make decisions for oneself is rather different to writing the directive, this should be treated separately from the common understanding of an advance directive. Again, it is not always easy to separate this out in the research.

A common criticism of advance directives is that the person is unable to consider all the circumstances in which the directive might need to apply. Thus a decision made in the past may not always suit current circumstances. One way round this is to understand the person's values and history, and base a decision on that. This involves taking what is usually referred to as a values history or narrative.

Where another person is involved in making the decision, particularly as proxy, there is the question of whether the criterion for the decision is substituted judgement or in the patient's (person's) best interest.

Substituted judgement and best interest

'Substituted judgement' is usually contrasted with 'best interest'. Substituted judgement is taken to mean that the agent (proxy, guardian) makes a decision based on what they believe the person themself would choose were they able (capable, competent) in the same situation. Best interest, in contrast, requires the agent to make the decision based on what is likely to achieve the best outcome for the person or best promote their well-being. Many medical decisions use the best interest standard: 'it is in the patient's best interest to take a medication they do not want as it will promote their well-being'; 'it is in a person's best interest to prevent/treat a suicide attempt as living is preferable to dying'. 'Well-being' is usually determined as continued living, as symptom-free as possible, even if the patient appears to believe otherwise.

'Least restrictive alternative' has also been used as criteria for assuming what is in the patient's best interest. The Millan Committee, in reviewing the mental health law in Scotland, took the view that being treated in the community was, by definition, less restrictive than being treated in hospital (Scottish Executive 2001) although not all patients agreed with this view (Atkinson 2006). A somewhat different approach to least restrictive alternative was the suggestion that following a patient's wishes as laid out in an advance directive would be, by definition, the least restrictive alternative, as it followed the person's choice (Atkinson and Garner 2002).

If respecting autonomy is to be truly prioritised as central to medical ethics then, by the same token, following an advance directive must be the decision in the person's best interest as this is the option which most respects autonomy. This would seem to be supported by the guidance given by the Department of Health (2001b) which indicated that best interests are not narrowly defined only as medical interests, but include: 'Values and preferences when competent, their psychological health, well-being, quality of life, relationships with family or other carers, spiritual and religious welfare and their own (i.e. the patient's) financial interests' (p.12).

Best interest is the assumption behind the state's power of *parens patriae*. This originated in the power of the King to act as guardian to his subjects who were incompetent and to promote their interests. Although it is invoked as a rationale for involuntary commitment and treatment it could be argued that its legitimacy has been lost where a mental health act allows for involuntary commitment and treatment of competent persons.

Substituted judgements are deemed to promote autonomy, basing the decision on what the patient would do in the circumstances. In this respect advance directives can be seen as a form of substituted decision-making, with the capable or well person making an advance substituted decision for the incapable or ill person.

In encouraging substituted decision-making, the proxy needs to consider the person's values and what decision the person would make, rather than the decision they would make for themself or based on their values. By doing this the guilt which often accompanies and complicates surrogate decisions, particularly in terminal illness, may decrease (Lang and Quill 2004).

Doing this is, however, by no means easy. It requires not just a good under-standing of the patient's values, wishes, preferences and goals, which may not be consistent, but also a good understanding of the current situation, the various alternatives for intervention, and the possible outcomes, side-effects and other consequences. This, in itself, is likely to be unachievable.

There is a further problem outlined by Baergen (1995a, 1995b). He sug-gested there are a number of 'non-values' of the person which can inappropriately influence a substituted judgement. These include:

> Distorted views of the world, of self, and of the future that are characteristic of depression; fear, denial of a serious illness; compulsive compliance; bias against health care providers...; the conviction that God will effect a miraculous cure (or the conviction that illness is a divine punishment); and the conviction that new medical advances will soon provide a cure (p.33).

Distinguishing the non-value aspect of some of these will be difficult, but necessary, to arrive at a decision which reflects values. Fear of pain may thus reflect an underlying value of living a pain-free life and may thus legitimately drive a substituted decision. Fear may often, however, be temporary or related to transient experience or based on a misunderstanding or lack of information.

Fear of surgery, for example, may be deemed to be fairly rational based on anxieties about anaesthetic and surgical complications, post-operative pain, loss of dignity and privacy as a consequence of hospital treatment, and so on. For most people, however, this will not stop them having life-saving or life-enhanc-ing surgery if the underlying values of continuing to live or enhancing quality of life are more important. A substituted judgement would have to be based on the core value rather than take account of temporary fear. Making judgements for another about not wanting electro-convulsive therapy (ECT), for example, thus need careful analysis to ensure this supports an underlying value of principle, rather than a natural fear of an intervention which may conflict with a core value.

Baergen (1995a, 1995b) suggested a revised version of the substituted judgement standard using a 'practical syllogism' which only takes account of 'statements of the patient's goals and values' and 'descriptions of the medical cir-cumstances'. All the confounding factors detailed above would then be ignored. He, and others (Smith and Nunn 1995), acknowledged that this does not make understanding the patient's core values any easier. Indeed Smith and Nunn argued that 'the luxury of certainty is not possible'. They go so far as to ask: 'Why does anyone believe that an individual really knows what he or she would want in any given medical situation?' (p.186). Agreeing that certainty is 'not available' Baergen (1995b) nevertheless argued that his revised version offered a greater degree of confidence in the judgement.

Although outwith the scope of this book the consideration of how substituted judgement might be involved in those with severe retardation who have never been competent helps clarify the type of decisions taken. This has been described as a 'legal fiction' by a court in Massachusetts in respect of a 33-year-old woman with severe mental retardation, Canavan's disease and in a persistent vegetative state. Martyn (1994), however, preferred to describe it as a 'fallacy' '…that someone other than this severely impaired patient could be trusted to fathom her intent, which she herself was never capable of grasping or expressing' (p.198).

Concerned that the court had, in fact, used its own, rather than substituted, judgement, which left the woman 'vulnerable to judicially sanctioned abuse', Martyn proposed a 'hybrid "best respect" legal standard':

> Best respect can be understood as a decision-making standard that rejects any result as inevitable, identifies a group of persons best able to collect the most relevant information concerning objective medical fact and subjective moral voice, and requires this group to meet with each other to maintain focus and correct misunderstanding (p.203).

This approach, she argued, means that even after careful and detailed consideration, with no further inquiry possible, the surrogate decision-maker can be sure that the patient has been respected as an individual rather than the sense that a 'rigid legal doctrine has been met'.

Proxy decision-making

Proxy decision-making is being treated here as something separate from an advance directive for two reasons. First, the decision to appoint a proxy and the issues involved in handing over decision-making to another person are different from a person making a statement of their wishes in future situations. Second, although in some jurisdictions, such as much of the United States, appointing a proxy or substitute decision-maker is incorporated into making an advance directive, this is not the case in other areas such as Britain. Even where proxies are supported, the law may specifically prevent them making certain decisions in relation to mental health treatment.

It is not always possible to separate these two reasons. Thus Swartz et al.'s (2006) comment that a health care power of attorney 'is the common form of PAD [psychiatric advance directive] (and the most commonly accepted by clinicians)' does not apply in, for example, Scotland. Furthermore, their reported views of patients on PADs might also not apply, as they suggest it might not to 'patients who wish to memorialise treatment refusal' and who do not want to appoint a proxy.

Although there may be different views on whether a proxy decision-maker is acting as substituted judgement or on best interests, the person appointing a proxy should understand what their local law says. In general if a person's wishes are unclear it is likely that the law will expect the person to act in the patient's best interests. Thus the law in Idaho, for example, states that where an agent does not know the patient's wishes 'the agent has a duty to act in what the agent believes to be the best interest of the principal' (Title 66.606 (c)). The law in Wisconsin is similar.

Whatever the law says, the proxy decision-maker will be able to act most appropriately the more they understand the wishes and intentions of the person for whom they are acting. If this is the case then the question must arise as to how well the proxy understands the decisions the patient would have made or the reasoning they may have used to reach such decisions.

There are no studies examining this in mental illness, but some understanding can be gained from studies in other areas. Research with people who are chronically ill, elderly and other seriously ill patients showed that family members were not very good at predicting or making the same judgements as ill family members (Ditto *et al.* 2001; Fried, Bradley and Towle 2003; Hare, Pratt and Nelson 1992; Pruchno *et al.* 2006; Seckler *et al.* 1991; Suhl *et al.* 1994; Tsevat *et al.* 1995; Upadya *et al.* 2002). A recent systematic review (Shalowitz, Garrett-Meyer and Wendler 2006) which collectively analysed over 19,500 patient-surrogate responses found that in one-third of cases the surrogates incorrectly identified the patient's end-of-life treatment preferences. This is a non-trivial number for such an important decision.

Not all studies, however, are so negative and Tomlinson *et al.* (1990) suggested that relatives were able to make judgements in a clinical scenario which came closer to the elderly person's judgement when specifically asked to make a substituted judgement than to their 'best recommendation'. The problem is compounded when the decision-making capacity of the surrogate is itself in question and where there are possible alternative surrogates (Bramstedt 2003). A study comparing family surrogates with physicians' views about elderly outpatients' treatment preferences in different scenarios found that, overall, relatives' judgements were more accurate than physicians' judgements (Coppola *et al.* 2001). Providing the physician with an advance directive had no effect on primary care physicians but did help hospital-based physicians to whom the patient was unknown.

Where there is no designated proxy, clinicians may involve relatives in decisions about care and treatment, particularly in relation to end-of-life scenarios. Although a number of relatives may be involved, the law will normally determine a hierarchy, usually spouse, adult children, parents. Lang and Quill (2004) outlined the form the discussion should usefully take, noting that the best understanding of the patient's values is not necessarily that of the next-of-kin. The difficulty of inferring values in unexpected situations is explored in a novel taking an extreme and rare scenario of a woman in a persistent vegetative state who is found to be pregnant, and follows the family discussions to reach some sort of consensus (McHaffie 2005).

Although it would seem advisable for anyone appointing a proxy decision-maker to discuss matters with the person they are naming, it is not always clear that this happens. The named person in Scotland is not a proxy decision-maker but will be involved in the legislative process, and the Scottish Executive (2004) nevertheless gives clear advice that the role and types of decisions should be discussed with the person before they are appointed. The National Empowerment Centre in the USA also offers good advice on choosing a health care agent (Fisher 2006).

Another issue which requires consideration is the freedom of the person to choose the most appropriate proxy. Particular family ties or obligations may mean that it is difficult, for example, not to appoint a spouse, although the person may prefer an adult child. The issue of family members involved in the process under mental health legislation has received little attention, but where it has the pressures and problems have been outlined (Atkinson 2006; Rapaport 2004, 2005), although positive aspects are noted (Taylor, Laurie and Geddes 1996).

Concern has been expressed that many people with severe mental illness may not have anyone they can ask to be proxy, or who they would trust in this role. This is reported by some patients themselves:

> I think I was very lucky to have a brother who could act as my health care proxy but I don't think many other survivors are that lucky and I think more should be done to help people get other people in their lives so they can advocate for them when they might need it (Bazelon Centre for Mental Health Law undated).

In the study by Swanson *et al.* (2006b), however, of a total of 153 advance directives made, 118 (77%) involved the appointment of a proxy. The authors do not report on whether there were problems in finding or appointing a power of attorney. Since in North Carolina advance instructions can also be made (which do not require a proxy), not having an available person does not prevent a person making an advance directive. This is not the case in all states.

Finally everyone needs to understand the role and powers of a proxy, whether appointed by the person in a power of attorney or appointed for an incapacitated person by the courts. A study in Quebec considering consent for both treatment and research with incapable adults showed knowledge varied not only between patient, carer, researcher and members of the research ethics boards but also between scenarios. Thus although knowledge was good for competent and legally represented patients in relation to treatment it was particularly poor among patients and carers in relation to consent for research (Bravo *et al.* 2003).

Joint crisis plans

Joint crisis plans fall into the middle ground between professionally led plans and advance directives. In a study which seems to use joint crisis plans and advance agreements synonymously Flood *et al.* (2006) describe their aim as 'to reach agreement between the service users and clinical team through negotiation and consensus building, facilitated by a third party' (p.729). This described a process aim as much as an outcome and not all joint crisis plans will involve an independent facilitator. Outcome aims will face some of the problems outlined earlier for advance directives though, since they have to be agreed with the team providing the service, they are likely to be closely aligned to their goals. Many of these, though, such as avoiding coercion through use of mental health legislation, are likely to be supported by patients. Reducing time in hospital may be supported by many, but not necessarily all patients, but for professionals may be linked to reducing service costs as much as quality of life outcomes. The cost savings described by Flood *et al.* (2006) may make them attractive to service managers.

A potential difference between joint crisis plans and advance directives is when they are invoked. The crisis plan, as it says, comes into being when the person is 'in crisis', a state they may well recognise, but before they would be judged legally incapable (or possibly even clinically incompetent). It is in that grey area that people are confused, not necessarily thinking clearly and that to be presented with former choices and decisions may be helpful. The lack of a clear distinction in both research and conception means it is difficult to separate them in terms of research evidence and so they have been incorporated in previous chapters.

Although one study (Sutherby *et al.* 1999) showed that patients preferred to make a crisis plan jointly rather than independently, in other studies the support of a member of staff (independent or not) is taken for granted and provided for in the design and it is not clear that this would be the patient's choice.

Joint crisis plans would seem to have much to offer, although they are unlikely to meet the needs of those who want an independent voice and a self-initiated plan or choices to which staff will not, or cannot, agree.

Values history

A 'values history' is a somewhat different approach to forward planning, although it could usefully be consolidated with the others. Rather than addressing specific scenarios the person recounts what is important to them, both as values to live by and intended outcomes. This allows others, whether the care team or an appointed proxy, to make decisions based on their understanding of the person. This goes beyond the standard cultural notes made regarding religion or dietary preferences, such as vegetarianism. It is a way of helping to ensure a substituted judgement is just that. It does not take the place of a clinician having a good, personal understanding of a patient, nor should such a relationship preclude the need for a written values history. It has a specific purpose in guiding decisions when the person is unable so to do.

To this end the range of the values history should be fairly extensive. Not all versions take in sufficient breadth, with a focus on treatment preferences with no indication of how these are related to general medical condition or overall treatment goals (Doukas and Gorenflo 1993; Doukas and McCullough 1994). Peters and Chiverton (2003) described it as a written questionnaire. This limited approach still persists. Das and Mulley (2005) suggested taking an 'ethics history' from patients who are not seriously ill to help manage any subsequent medical crisis. The questions they proposed, however, are very limited and related more to practical issues, including organ donation, rather than understanding a person's ethical beliefs and reasoning.

A good, wide ranging values history may be particularly important where there is little personal knowledge. Bernstein (2006) noted, 'The mental health system often knows very little about the individuals it serves, even its long-standing consumers. Clinical relationships in public mental health, both in hospital and community contexts, tend to be quite transient' (p.403).

Although not values histories, the reasons given for making particular decisions encouraged in some jurisdictions or by some forms, incorporate elements of their purpose. They allow the treating team to understand what is important to the person. Without such an understanding even a fairly detailed advance directive may not allow for the spirit of the directive to be followed if the detail cannot be provided. Thus the detailed requests given by Dace (2001) included being allowed to spend time alone reading, being able to eat alone and being given art material 'to use privately'. She also includes 'at least 20 minutes a day walking in a quiet location, accompanied if necessary'. There is also a statement that 'when distressed I am extremely sensitive to noise' followed by a request for a quiet, calm environment. Quietness would thus seem to be important, but it is not clear whether privacy (or being alone) is also an important issue or whether this is a way of ensuring quiet.

Some people would argue that as they have a right to their choice of accepting treatment or not they should not have to explain their reasons. Although they might be right in this assertion, explaining important values allows those who have to respond to the advance directive to follow its spirit, even if they cannot always comply with the detail.

CHAPTER 15

Conclusion: The Way Forward

Recently the interest in advance directives in mental health has grown, not only in terms of research but also in terms of legislative activity. It is not always clear, though, that clinical involvement has grown at the same rate.

In legislative terms Scotland has led the way in Britain by introducing advance statements within the Mental Health (Care and Treatment) (Scotland) Act 2003 whereas the idea did not find favour with the Government in England and Wales. A number of states in the USA have introduced specific legislation and in other places, including Australia and parts of Europe, interest is growing as mental health laws are reviewed.

The law is variable. Although progress has been made with specific laws allowing mental health advance directives, there is still some concern that there is discrimination. Laws being written less favourably or enforced less often (or, conversely, over-written more often) than most covering physical health. The thorny question of the relationship between an advance directive and status as an involuntary patient persists. Tackling this involves working with politicians, legislators, judges and tribunal members. In the USA the Protection and Advocacy for Individuals with Mental Illness Program sets out to educate state legislators and judges along with clinicians and service users (Priaulx 2003).

Although more and more research studies are being published on all aspects of advance directives, from encouraging patients to make one to their enactment, at the moment most of this comes from the programme at Duke University in North Carolina. This work is impressive and helpful but it reflects one programme in one setting. To translate this into Britain may be less straightforward since there are differences in both the law on advance directives and the mental health acts. Many of the states in the USA require or expect the appointment of a proxy as part of making an advance directive. When the separate aspects of advance instruction and proxies are considered independently it is clear that patients in general like the idea of having a proxy or surrogate. In Britain there is no provision for the appointment of a proxy (apart from incapacity/capacity legislation) in the same way that there is in the USA.

There is no direct comparison between advance directives in the two countries. Since the legislation itself differs, in terms of requirements for making an advance directive and provisions given against over-rides, or allowing these, attitudes to advance directives will differ as will their use and impact. The relationship of advance directives with criteria commitment is central.

Similarly there are differences in mental health acts between the UK and the USA, including criteria for commitment and compulsory treatment and these might make patients view having an advance directive differently. Scotland is unusual in having advance statements embedded in its Mental Health Act rather than separate legislation – legislation, furthermore, which means that the advance statement is intended to come into play at the time of compulsory treatment. The mental health laws also differ in their approach to compulsory treatment and the use of the least restrictive alternative. In parts of the USA sedation and restraint are more commonly used than in Britain (where medication is more common) and appears as a specific category in some of the reforms. Avoiding this may be important for patients and may make them more willing to give medication preferences. Conversely, it may make everyone clearer about the positive consequences of treatment refusal and in some cases make this easier to accept. Direct consideration of sedation and restraint does not appear to have taken place in Britain.

The impact of the different health care systems is also unclear. It would appear that most of the research in the USA is within public psychiatric hospitals. Many of the people to whom advance directives are likely to have most relevance are also unlikely to have private medical insurance. Greater understanding of insurers and private facilities' views of psychiatric advance directives would be valuable. In the USA advance directives usually allow the person to specify (within limits) what facility they would use, but this is not something considered in Britain.

To many, the disappointing uptake of advance directives outwith research settings should not have come as a surprise. Following the introduction of the Patient Self-Determination Act, uptake of advance directives in physical health was not as extensive as had been anticipated. What has become clear is that making an advance directive, of any kind, is not an easy procedure for most patients and may need to be completed over a period of time. It is also clear that this process is greatly enhanced by having someone work with the patient to make the advance directive. It is not altogether clear that this needs to be someone independent of the treatment team.

The other major barrier to patients making an advance directive seems to be a belief that it will not make a difference to how they are treated. Many patients will not see the point in making an advance directive if it is automatically trumped by the Mental Health Act. The legal provisions for allowing advance directives to be over-ridden by clinicians in other circumstances only adds to the sense of pointlessness.

The lack of enthusiasm from different professional groups, but probably especially from psychiatrists, contributes to both the above problems. Clinicians are not actively seeking to promote advance directives, so patients do not know about them and do not get help in making them. This would suggest that at least as much energy must go into educating professionals and motivating them as is needed in promoting advance directives to patients.

Some of the clinicians' anxiety might be allayed if they were involved in the process, and for most patients this seems to be a positive move. Those who want them to be entirely independent will not be prohibited from doing this (unless the only option is an advance agreement or joint crisis plan). The evidence that very few patients refuse all medication should also be reassuring to those who fear that promoting advance directives will lead to large numbers of untreated and untreatable patients.

As more advance directives are made there will be more evidence on the outcomes. This is likely to include what happens to the few patients who refuse all medication. Although the evidence is most likely to come from case studies (at least at first) this will still allow commonalities to be highlighted and the implications assessed. More research, from a wider range of services and settings, would also be helpful as would a wider understanding of what might be appropriate outcomes.

Research need not be in the form of randomised controlled trials. Indeed, this might not be the best way forward for something which is not, in itself, an intervention. It may be that focusing on outcomes from the patient's perspective would be advantageous, as might a different methodological approach altogether, moving, for example, into translational research. Another possible approach, adapted from business and engineering, would be to develop methodology using the framework of continuous improvement methodology. This would help to locate the research in real settings, with all the clinical and resource constraints that this implies.

More fundamental questions may need to be raised about the philosophy behind advance directives in mental health, especially 'What are they for?' Many of the early assumptions about supporting autonomy may still stand, but will be placed in a wider framework. Autonomy does not have to mean being independent. It could include having improved relationships between patients and clinicians, ensuring that communication is enhanced and that there is more appropriate sharing of ideas and making realistic choices, whether to preferred treatment or to the options and consequences of reduced treatment.

Advance statements can be seen as much as a tool for accepting responsibility as enhancing autonomy. Within a service framework which increasingly looks for

the participation of patients in their treatment and management, promoting this aspect may sit well with service providers and planners.

What would be unfortunate would be if the 'slow start', or the less than convincing evidence for clinical impact and use of services, were seen as a reason for not bothering with advance directives. The development of advance directives in mental health is facing challenges, but also opportunities. For them to be useful, for both patients and clinicians means both parties must be involved in the process of developing them into a workable tool, available for all who want them, and able to meet a variety of ends. The priority, however, is the people who make them and they must be included in this process. No matter how the outcome is measured it should focus on the patient – the service user – and not the services. Having an advance directive must remain an individual choice for each patient and not become a routine form to fill in with a few prescribed choices. Whatever else, autonomy must remain at their heart.

References

Amador, X.F., Flaum, M., Andreasen, N.C., Strauss, D.H. *et al.* (1994) 'Awareness of illness in schizophrenia and schizoaffective mood disorder.' *Archives of General Psychiatry 51*, 826–836.

American Psychiatric Association's Task Force on Research Ethics (2006) 'Ethical principles and practice for research involving human participants with mental illness.' *Psychiatric Services 57*, 552–557.

Amering, M., Stastny, P., Hopper, P. (2005) 'Psychiatric advance directives: qualitative study of informed deliberations by mental health service users.' *British Journal of Psychiatry 186*, 247–252.

Anderson, N. (2003) 'Dr Jekyll's waiver of Mr Hyde's right to refuse medical treatment. Washington's new law authorizing mental health care advance directives needs additional protections.' *Washington Law Review 78*, 795–829.

Anonymous (2004) 'Psychiatric advance directives: a user's view.' *Psychiatric Bulletin 28*, 134.

Anthony, P., Crawford, P. (2000) 'Service user involvement in care planning: the mental health nurses' perspective.' *Journal of Psychiatry and Mental Health Nursing 7*, 425–434.

Appelbaum, P. (1994) *Almost a Revolution. Mental Health Law and the Limits of Change.* Oxford: Oxford University Press.

Appelbaum, P. (2004) 'Psychiatric advance directives and the treatment of committed patients.' *Psychiatric Services 55*, 751–763.

Appelbaum, P.S. (2006) 'Commentary: Psychiatric advance directives at the crossroads – when can PADs be overridden?' *Journal of the American Academy of Psychiatry and Law 43*, 395–397.

Appelbaum, P.S., Grisso, T., Frank, E., O'Donnell, S. *et al.* (1999) 'Competence of depressed patients for consent to research.' *American Journal of Psychiatry 156*, 1380–1384.

Appelbaum, P.S., Redlich, A. (2006) 'Impact of decisional capacity on the use of leverage to encourage treatment adherence.' *Community Mental Health Journal 42*, 121–130.

Atkinson, J.M. (1994) 'Community care and the new right.' *Journal of Mental Health 3*, 423–425.

Atkinson, J.M. (1996) 'The community of strangers: supervision and the new right.' *Health and Social Care in the Community 4*, 122–125.

Atkinson, J.M. (2004) 'Ulysses' crew or Circe? – The implications of advance directives in mental health for psychiatrists.' *Psychiatric Bulletin 28*, 3–4.

Atkinson, J.M. (2006) *Private and Public Protection: The New Mental Health Regime.* Edinburgh: Dunedin Academic Press.

Atkinson, J.M., Coia, D.A. (1989) 'Responsibility to carers – an ethical dilemma.' *Psychiatric Bulletin 12*, 602–604.

Atkinson, J.M., Coia, D.A. (1995) *Families Coping with Schizophrenia. A Practical Guide to Family Groups.* Chichester: John Wiley.

Atkinson, J.M., Garner, H.C. (2002) 'Least restrictive alternative – advance statements and the new mental health legislation.' *Psychiatric Bulletin 26,* 246–247.

Atkinson, J.M., Garner, H.C., Gilmour, W.H. (2004) 'Models of advance directives in mental health care: Stakeholder views.' *Social Psychiatry and Psychiatric Epidemiology 39,* 673–680.

Atkinson, J.M., Garner, H.C., Patrick, H., Stuart, S. (2003a) 'Issues in the development of advance directives in mental health care.' *Journal of Mental Health 12,* 463–474.

Atkinson, J.M., Garner, H.C., Stuart, S., Patrick, H. (2003b) 'The development of potential models of advance directives in mental health care.' *Journal of Mental Health 12,* 575–584.

Atkinson, J.M., MacPherson, K. (2001) 'Patient's advocacy: the development of a service at the State Hospital, Carstairs.' *Journal of Mental Health 10,* 589–596.

Atkinson, J.M., Reilly, J., Garner, H.C., Patterson, L.E. (2005) *Review of Literature Relating to Mental Health Legislation.* Edinburgh: Scottish Executive.

Backlar, P. (1994) *Can I plan now for the treatment I would want if I were in crisis? A Guide to Oregon's Declaration for Mental Health Treatment.* State of Oregon Office of Mental Health Services, Mental Health and Developmental Disability Services Division.

Backlar, P. (1995) 'The longing for order: Oregon's medical advance directive for mental health treatment.' *Community Mental Health Journal 31,* 103–108.

Backlar, P. (1997) 'Anticipatory planning for end-of-life care is not quite like anticipatory planning for psychiatric treatment.' *Community Mental Health Journal 33,* 261–268.

Backlar, P. (1998) 'Advance directives for subjects of research who have fluctuating cognitive impairments due to psychiatric disorders (such as schizophrenia).' *Community Mental Health Journal 34,* 229–240.

Backlar, P., McFarland, B.H. (1996) 'A survey on the use of advance directives for mental health treatment in Oregon.' *Psychiatric Services 47,* 1387–1389.

Backlar, P., McFarland, B.H. (1998) 'Oregon's advance directive for mental health treatment: Implications for policy.' *Administration and Policy in Mental Health 25,* 609–618.

Backlar, P., McFarland, B.H., Swanson, J.W., Mahler, J. (2001) 'Consumer, provider and informal caregiver opinions on psychiatric advance directives.' *Administration and Policy in Mental Health 28,* 427–441.

Baergen, R. (1995a) 'Revising the substituted judgement standard.' *Journal of Clinical Ethics 6,* 30–38.

Baergen, R. (1995b) 'Commentary: surrogates and uncertainty.' *Journal of Clinical Ethics 6,* 372–377.

Barnes, M., Shardlow, P. (1997) 'From passive recipient to active citizen: participation in mental health user groups.' *Journal of Mental Health 6,* 289–300.

Barrett, A., Roques, T., Small, M., Smith, R.D. (2006) 'How much will Herceptin really cost?' *British Medical Journal 333,* 118–1120.

Bazelon Centre for Mental Health Law (undated) *Power in Planning. Self-determination through psychiatric advance directives.* www.bazelon.org/issues/advanceddirectives/publications

Bean, P. (2001) *Mental Disorder and Community Safety.* Basingstoke, Hampshire: Palgrave.

Beeforth, M., Conlan, E., Graley, R. (1994) *Have We Got Views For You: User Evaluation of Care Management.* London: Sainsbury Centre for Mental Health.

Benn, S. (1989) *A Theory of Freedom.* Cambridge: Cambridge University Press.

Berg, J.W. (1996) 'Legal and ethical complexities of consent with cognitively impaired subjects: proposed guidelines.' *Archives of General Psychiatry 54*, 18–35.

Bernstein, R. (2006) 'Commentary: The climate for physician adherence to psychiatric advance directives.' *Journal of the American Academy for Psychiatry and the Law 34*, 402–405.

Berofsky, B. (1995) *Liberation from Self. A Theory of Personal Autonomy.* Cambridge: Cambridge University Press.

Bhui, K., Aubin, A., Strathdee, G. (1998) 'Making a reality of user involvement in community mental health services.' *Psychiatric Bulletin 22*, 8–11.

Biegler, P., Stewart, C., Savulescuh, J., Shene, L. (2000) 'Determining the validity of advance directives.' *Medical Journal of Australia 172*, 545–548.

Bindman, J., Beck, A., Glover, G., Thornicroft, G. *et al.* (1999) 'Evaluating health policy in England. Care programme approach and supervision registers.' *British Journal of Psychiatry 175*, 327–330.

Bleuler, E. (1911/1950) *The Fundamental Symptoms of Dementia Praecox or the Group of Schizophrenias.* Transl. Zinkin, J. New York: International Universities Press.

Boardman, J. (2005) 'New services for old – An overview of mental health policy.' In Bell, A., Lindley, P. (eds) *Beyond the Water Towers. The Unfinished Revolution in Mental Health Services 1985–2005.* London: Sainsbury Centre for Mental Health.

Bonnie, R.J. (1997) 'Research with cognitively impaired subjects; unfinished business in the regulation of human research.' *Archives of General Psychiatry 54*, 105–111.

Bourgeois, W. (1995) *Persons. What Philosophers Say About You.* Waterloo, Ontario: Wilfred Laurier University Press.

Bowl, R. (1996) 'Involving service users in mental health services: social service departments and the NHS and Community Care Act.' *Journal of Mental Health 5*, 287–303.

Bramstedt, K.A. (2003) 'Questioning the decision-making capacity of surrogates.' *Internal Medicine Journal 33*, 257–259.

Bravo, G., Paquet, M., Dubois, M-F. (2003) 'Knowledge of the legislation governing proxy consent to treatment and research.' *Journal of Medical Ethics 29*, 44–50.

Brennan, R.P. (1992) *Dictionary of Scientific Literacy.* New York: John Wiley.

Brock, D.W. (1991) 'Trumping advance directives.' *Hastings Centre Report 21*, S5–S6.

Brock, D.W. (1998) 'Commentary on the time frame of preferences, dispositions, and the validity of advance directives for the mentally ill.' *Philosophy, Psychiatry and Psychology 5*, 251–253.

Brown, S.J., Lumley, J. (1998) 'Communication and decision-making in labour: do birth plans make a difference?' *Health Expectations 1*, 106–116.

Burgess, S.L. (1998) 'Commentary on the time frame of preferences, dispositions, and the validity of advance directives for the mentally ill.' *Philosophy, Psychiatry and Psychology 5*, 255–258.

Campbell, P. (1999) 'Written in Advance.' *OpenMind* Sept/Oct 24.

Campbell, P. (2005) 'From little acorns – the mental health service user movement.' In Bell, A., Lindley, P. (eds) *Beyond the Water Towers. The Unfinished Revolution in Mental Health Services 1985–2005.* London: Sainsbury Centre for Mental Health.

Carlile, A. (2005) 'Legislation to Law: Rubicon or Styx.' *Journal of Mental Health Law 13*, 107–209.

Carpenter, J., Schneider, J., McNiven, F., Brandon, T. *et al.* (2004) 'Integration and targeting of community care for people with severe and enduring mental health problems; users' experiences of the Care Programme Approach and Care Management.' *British Journal of Social Work 34*, 313–333.

Cerminara, K.L. (2003) 'Advance directives in the United States'. *Summons* Summer, 8–9.

Chadwick, E. (1842) *Report on the Sanitary Conditions of the Labouring Population of Great Britain.* Reprinted 1965, edited by M.W. Flinn. Edinburgh: Edinburgh University Press.

Chadwick, P.K. (1997) *Schizophrenia: The Positive Perspective. In Search of Dignity for Schizophrenic People.* London: Routledge.

Chief Medical Officer (2001) *Expert Patients Programme.* London: Department of Health.

Copeland, M.E. (2004) *Advance Directives.* NAMI SCC Website: www.namiscc.org/recovery/2004/AdvanceDirectives.htm

Coppola, K.M., Ditto, P.H., Danks, J.H., Smucker, W. (2001) 'Accuracy of primary care and hospital-based physicians' predictions of elderly outpatients' treatment preferences with and without advance directives.' *Archives of Internal Medicine 161*, 431–440.

Corrigan, P.W., Watson, A.C., Heyrman, M.L., Warpinski, A. *et al.* (2005) 'Structural stigma in State legislation.' *Psychiatric Services 56*, 557–563.

Crossley, N. (1998) 'Transforming the mental health field: the early history of the National Association for Mental Health.' *Sociology of Health and Illness 20*, 458–488.

Crossley, N. (1999) 'Fish, field, habitus and madness: the first wave mental health movement in Great Britain.' *British Journal of Sociology 50*, 647–670.

Crossley, M.L., Crossley, N. (2001) 'Patients' voices, social movements and the habitus; how psychiatric survivors "speak out".' *Social Science and Medicine 52*, 1477–1489.

Cuca, R. (1993) 'Ulysses in Minnesota: first steps towards a self-binding psychiatric advance statute.' *Cornell Law Review 78*, 1152–1186.

Culver, C., Gert, B. (1981) 'The morality of involuntary hospitalisation.' In Spicker, J.M., Healy, J.R., Engelhart, J.R. (eds) *The Law Medicine Relations: A Philosophical Exploration.* Boston: Reidel.

Curran, C., Grimshaw, C. (1999) 'Advance directives.' *OpenMind Sept/Oct*, 24.

Dace, E. (2001) 'A cat among the pigeons.' *Mental Health Today Nov*, 29–31.

Das, A.K., Mulley, G.P. (2005) 'The value of an ethics history?' *Journal of the Royal Society of Medicine 98*, 262–266.

Davis, J.K. (2002) 'The concept of precedent autonomy'. *Bioethics 16*, 114-133.

Davis, J.K. (2004) 'Precedent autonomy and subsequent consent.' *Ethical Theory and Moral Practice 7*, 267–291.

Dawson, J., King, M., Papageorgiou, A., Davidson, O. (2001) 'Legal pitfalls of psychiatric research.' *British Journal of Psychiatry 178*, 67–70.

Dawson, J., Szmukler, G. (2006) 'Fusion of mental health and incapacity legislation.' *British Journal of Psychiatry 188*, 504–509.

Degen, K., Nasper, E. (1996) *Return from Madness. Psychotherapy with People Taking the New Anti-Psychotic Medications and Emerging from Severe, Lifelong and Disabling Schizophrenia.* Northwale, New Jersey: Jason Aronson.

Department for Constitutional Affairs (2003) *Making Decisions: Helping People who have Difficulty in Deciding for Themselves. Planning Ahead. A Guide for People Who Wish to Prepare for Possible Future Incapacity.* London: Department for Constitutional Affairs.

Department of Health (1990) *Caring for People. The Care Programme Approach for People with a Mental Illness Referred to Specialist Mental Health Services.* Joint Health/Social Services Circular C(90)23/LASSL(90)11.

Department of Health (1995) *Building Bridges. A Guide to the Arrangements for Interagency Working for the Care and Protection of Severely Mentally Ill People.* London: The Stationery Office.

Department of Health (1998) *Modernising Mental Health Services.* London: HMSO.

Department of Health (1999) *Review of the Mental Health Act 1983 (Richardson Report).* London: HMSO.

Department of Health (2001a) *Good Practice in Consent Implementation Guide: Consent for Examination or Treatment.* London: HMSO.

Department of Health (2001b) *Reference Guide to Consent for Examination or Treatment.* London: HMSO.

Department of Health (2004) *Choose and Book – Patients' Choice of Hospital and Booked Appointments.* London: HMSO.

Department of Health (2005) *Government Response to the Report of the Joint Committee on the Draft Mental Health Bill 2004,* cm6624. London: HMSO.

Derbyshire Mental Health Services NHS Trust (2003) *Advance Directive Policy.* www.derbyshire mentalhealthservices.nhs.uk

Derbyshire Mental Health Services NHS Trust (2004) *Guides for People Making an Advance Directive.* www.derbyshirementalhealthservices.nhs.uk

Ditto, P.H., Danks, J.H., Smucker, W.D., Bookwala, J. *et al.* (2001) 'Advance directives as acts of communication.' *Archives of Internal Medicine 161,* 421–430.

Dix, D. (1843) *On Behalf of the Insane Poor: Report to the Legislature of Massachusetts of January 1843.* Reprinted 1971 New York: Arno Press.

Doukas, D., Gorenflo, D. (1993) 'Analysing the values history: An evaluation of patients' medical values and advance directive.' *Journal of Clinical Ethics 4,* 41–45.

Doukas, D., McCullough, L. (1994) 'The values history; the evaluation of the patient's values and advance directives.' *Journal of Family Practice 32,* 145–153.

Doyal, L., Sheather, J. (2005) 'Mental health legislation should respect decision making capacity. *British Medical Journal 331,* 1467–1471.

Dresser, R. (1982) 'Ulysses and the psychiatrists: A legal policy analysis of the voluntary commitment contract.' *Harvard Civil Rights–Civil Liberties Law Review 16,* 833–835.

Dresser, R. (1984) 'Bound to treatment: The Ulysses contract.' *Hastings Centre Report 14,* 13–16.

Dresser, R. (1994) 'Advance directives; implications for policy.' *Hastings Centre Report 24, special supplement,* S2–S5.

Dresser, R. (1996) 'Mentally disabled research subjects: the enduring policy issues.' *Journal of the American Medical Association 276,* 67–72.

Dresser, R. (1998) 'Commentary on the time frame, preference, dispositions and the validity of advance directives for the mentally ill.' *Philosophy, Psychology and Psychiatry 5,* 247–249.

Duke University (2003) 'NIMH funds $1.98 million study to examine effectiveness of advance directives for patients with mental illness.' www.dukemednews.org/news/article.php?id_7036

Dunlap, J.A. (2000–1) 'Mental health advance directives: having one's say?' *Kentucky Law Journal 39,* 327–386.

Dunn, S. (1999) *Creating Accepting Communities; Report of the MIND Inquiry into Social Exclusion and Mental Health Problems.* London: MIND.

Dyer, C. (2006) 'Third time lucky.' *British Medical Journal 333,* 1090.

Dyer, C. (2007) 'Government suffers its first defeat over Mental Health Bill.' *British Medical Journal 334*, 113.

Eastman, N. (1994) 'Mental Health Law: civil liberties and the principles of reciprocity.' *British Medical Journal 308*, 43–45.

Eastman, N. (1998) 'Commentary on the time frame preference, dispositions and the validity of advance directives for the mentally ill.' *Philosophy, Psychology and Psychiatry 5*, 259–261.

Eastman, N. (1999) 'Public health psychiatry or crime prevention?' *British Medical Journal 318*, 549–551.

Eastman, N., Peay, J. (eds) (1999) *Law Without Enforcement. Integrating Mental Health and Justice.* Oxford: Hart.

Elbogen, E., Swartz, M.S., Van Dorn, R., Swanson, J.W. *et al.* (2006) 'Clinical decision making and views about psychiatric advance directives.' *Psychiatric Services 57*, 350–355.

Elliott, C. (1996) *The Rules of Insanity. Moral Responsibility and the Mentally Ill Offender.* Albany: State University of New York Press.

Elsler, J. (1979) *Ulysses and the Sirens. Studies in Rationality and Irrationality.* Cambridge: Cambridge University Press.

Emanuel, L.L. (2004) 'Advance directives and advancing age.' *Journal of the American Geriatric Society 52*, 641–642.

Fagerlin, A., Schneider, C.E. (2004) 'Enough: The failure of the living will.' *Hastings Centre Report 24*, 30–42.

Feinberg, J. (1970) *Doing and Deserving. Essays in the Theory of Responsibility.* Princeton, New Jersey: Princeton University Press.

Feinberg, J. (1986) *The Moral Limits of the Common Law. Vol 3. Harm to Self.* Oxford: Oxford University Press.

Fennell, P. (1996) *Treatment Without Consent. Law, Psychiatry and the Treatment of Mentally Disordered People since 1845.* London: Routledge.

Fennell, P. (2005) 'Protection! Protection! Protection! Déjà vu all over again. The Government response to the Parliamentary Scrutiny Committee.' *Journal of Mental Health Law 13*, 110–122.

Fisher, D. (2006) 'Making advance directives work for you.' Lawrence, Massachusetts, USA: National Empowerment Center. www.power2u.org/articles/selfhelp/directives_work

Flood, C., Byford, S., Henderson, C., Leese, M. *et al.* (2006) 'Joint crisis plans for people with psychosis: economic evaluation of a randomised controlled trial.' *British Medical Journal 333*, 729–732.

Ford, R., Beadsmoore, P., Norton, P., Cooke, A. *et al.* (1993) 'Developing case management for the long term mentally ill.' *Psychiatric Bulletin 17*, 409–411.

Ford, R., Rafferty, J., Ryan, P., Beadsmoore, A. *et al.* (1997) 'Intensive case management for people with serious mental illness: Site 2 – clinical and social outcomes.' *Journal of Mental Health 6*, 181–190.

Foti, M.E., Bartels, S.J., Merriman, M.P., Fletcher, K.E. *et al.* (2005a) 'Medical advance care planning for persons with serious mental illness.' *Psychiatric Services 56*, 576–584.

Foti, M.E., Bartels, S.J., Van Citters, A.D., Merriman, M.P. *et al.* (2005b) 'End-of-life treatment preferences of persons with serious mental illness.' *Psychiatric Services 56*, 585–591.

French, P.A. (1992) *Responsibility Matters.* Lawrence, Kansas: University Press of Kansas.

Fried, T.R., Bradley, E.H., Towle, V.R. (2003) 'Valuing the outcomes of treatment; do patients and their caregivers agree?' *Archives of Internal Medicine 163*, 2073–2078.

Gale, E., Grove, B. (2005) 'The social context for mental health.' In Bell, A., Lindley, P. (eds) *Beyond the Water Towers. The Unfinished Revolution in Mental Health Services 1985–2005.* London: Sainsbury Centre for Mental Health.

Gardner, S. (1993) *Irrationality and the Philosophy of Psychoanalysis.* Cambridge: Cambridge University Press.

Geller, J.L. (2000) 'The use of advance directives by persons with serious mental illness for psychiatric assessment.' *Psychiatric Quarterly 71,* 1–13.

Geller, J.L. (2003) 'Commentary (on Papageorgiou *et al.* 2002).' *Evidence-based Mental Health 6,* 89.

Giannini, A., Pessina, A., Tacchi, E.M. (2003) 'End-of-life decisions in intensive care units. Attitudes of physicians in an Italian urban setting.' *Intensive Care Medicine 29,* 1902–1910.

Goldman, H.H. (2005) 'A view from abroad.' In Bell, A., Lindley, P. (eds) *Beyond the Water Towers. The Unfinished Revolution in Mental Health Services 1985–2005.* London: Sainsbury Centre for Mental Health.

Gostin, L. (1975) *The Human Condition.* London: MIND.

Gray, J.E., Shone, M.A., Liddle, P.F. (in press) *Canadian Mental Health Law and Policy,* 2nd edition. Toronto: Butterworths.

Greco, P.J., Schulman, K.A., Lavizzo-Mourey, R., Hansen-Flaschen, J. (1991) 'The Patient Self-determination Act and the future of advance directives.' *Annals of Internal Medicine 115,* 639–643.

Griffiths, Sir R. (1988) *Community Care: Agenda for Action. A Report to the Secretary of State for Social Services by Sir Roy Griffiths.* London: HMSO.

Grisso, T., Appelbaum, P.S. (1995) 'The MacArthur Treatment Competence Study: III. Abilities of patients to consent to psychiatric and medical treatments.' *Law and Human Behaviour 19,* 149–174.

Grisso, T., Appelbaum, P.S. (1996) 'Values and limits of the MacArthur Treatment Competence Study.' *Psychology, Public Policy and Law 2,* 167–181.

Grisso, T., Appelbaum, P.S., Mulvey, E.P., Fletcher, K. (1995) 'The MacArthur Treatment Competence Study: II. Measures of abilities related to competence to consent to treatment.' *Law and Human Behaviour 19,* 127–148.

Gurevitz, H. (1977) 'Tarasoff: Protective privilege versus public peril.' *American Journal of Psychiatry 134,* 289–292.

Gutheil, T.G. (1980) 'In search of true freedom: drug refusal, involuntary medication and "rotting with your rights on".' American Journal of Psychiatry 137, 327–328.

Habermas, J. (1981) 'New social movements.' *Telos 48,* 33–37.

Halpern, A., Szmukler, G. (1997) 'Psychiatric advance directives; recognising autonomy and non-consensual treatment.' *Psychiatric Bulletin 21,* 8–9.

Halpern, D., Barnes, C. (2004) *Personal Responsibility and Changing Behaviour: the State of Knowledge and its Implications for Public Policy.* London Cabinet Office: Prime Minister's Strategy Unit.

Hamann, J., Cohen, R., Leucht, S., Kissling, W. (2005) 'Do patients with schizophrenia wish to be involved in decisions about their medical treatment.' *American Journal of Psychiatry 162,* 2382–2384.

Hare, J., Pratt, C., Nelson, C. (1992) 'Agreement between patients and their self-selected surrogates on difficult medical decisions.' *Archives of Internal Medicine 152,* 1058–1064.

Häyry, H. (1991) *The Limits of Medical Paternalism.* London: Routledge.

Häyry, M. (1994) *Liberal Utilitarianism and Applied Ethics.* London: Routledge.

Hayward, P., Bright, J.A. (1997) 'Stigma and mental illness: A review and critique.' *Journal of Mental Health 6*, 345–354.

Henderson, C., Flood, C., Leese, M., Thornicroft G. *et al.* (2004) 'Effect of joint crisis plans on use of compulsory treatment in psychiatry: single blind randomised controlled trial.' *British Medical Journal 329*, 136–139 (abridged version). www.bmj.com/cgi/content/full/329/7458/136 (full version)

Hildén, H-M., Louhiala, P., Palo, J. (2004) 'End of life decisions: attitudes of Finnish physicians.' *Journal of Medical Ethics 30*, 362–365.

Hoffman, D.E., Zimmerman, S.I., Tompkins, C.J. (1996) 'The dangers of directives or the false security of forms.' *Journal of Law and Medical Ethics 24*, 5–17.

Honberg, R.S. (2000) 'Advance directives.' *Journal of the National Association for Mental Illness 11*, 68–70. www.nami.org/content/contentgroups/Legal/Advance_directives.htm

Hooper, S.C., Vaughn, K.J., Tennant, C.C., Perz, J. (1996) 'Major depression and refusal of life-sustaining medical treatment in the elderly.' *Medical Journal of Australia 165*, 416–419.

House of Commons (1990) *The National Health Services and Community Care Act.* London: HMSO.

House of Lords and House of Commons Joint Committee on the Draft Mental Health Bill (2005) *Draft Mental Health Bill. Session 2004–5, Vol. 1.* London: HMSO.

Howell, T., Diamond, R., Winkler, D. (1982) 'Is there a case for voluntary commitment?' In Beauchamp, T., Walter, L. (eds) *Contemporary Issues in Bioethics.* Belmont, California: Wadsworth.

Inch, S. (1988) 'Birth plans and protocols.' *Journal of the Royal Society Medicine 81*, 12–22.

Jones, K. (1991) 'Law and mental health: sticks or carrots?' In Berrios, G.E., Freeman, H. (eds) *150 Years of British Psychiatry 1841–1991.* London: Gaskell.

Kamara, S.G., Peterson, P.D., Dennis, J.L. (1998) 'Prevalence of physical illness among psychiatric inpatients who die of natural causes.' *Psychiatric Services 49*, 788–793.

Kant, I. (1785/1969) *Groundwork of the Metaphysics of Morals.* Transl. Paton, H.J. *The Moral Law.* London: Hutchinson University Library.

Kennedy, A., Rogers, A., Gately, C. (2005) 'From patients to providers: prospects for self-care skills trainers in the National Health Service.' *Health and Social Care in the Community 13*, 431–440.

Keyserling, E.W., Glass, K., Kogan, S., Gauthier, S. (1995) 'Proposed guidelines for the participation of persons with dementia as research subjects.' *Perspectives in Biology and Medicine 38*, 319–362.

King, M., Papageorgiou, A., Dawson, J. (2003) 'How should advance statements be implemented? Authors' reply.' *British Journal of Psychiatry 182*, 549.

Kingdon, D.G., Turkington, D. (1994) 'The use of cognitive behavioural therapy and normalising rationale in schizophrenia.' *Journal of Nervous and Mental Disease 179*, 207–211.

Kingdon, D.G., Turkington, D. (2004) *Cognitive Therapy of Schizophrenia,* New York: Guilford Press.

Kitwood, T., Benson, S. (1995) *The New Culture of Dementia Care.* London: Hawker.

Kitwood, T., Bredin, K. (1992) 'Towards a theory of dementia care: personhood and well-being.' *Ageing and Society 12*, 269–287.

Kitzinger, S. (1992) 'Sheila Kitzinger's letter from England: Birth plans.' *Birth 19*, 36–37.

Kitzinger, S. (2000) *Rediscovering Birth.* New York: Pocket Books.

Kraeplin, E. (1896/1919) *Dementia Praecox and Paraphrenia.* Transl. Barclay, R.M. Edinburgh: E. and S. Livingstone.

Lambert, H. (2005) *Advance Medical Decision-Making in Long Term Care. Patient, Provider and Policy Perspectives.* Ontario, Canada: The Change Foundation. www.changefoundation.com

Lang, F., Quill, T. (2004) 'Making decisions with families at the end of life.' *American Family Physician 70,* 719–723.

Lawson, M., Strickland, C., Wolfson, P. (1999) 'User involvement in care planning. The Care Programme Approach (CPA) from the user's perspective.' *Psychiatric Bulletin 23,* 539–561.

Leff, J. (2001) 'Why is care in the community perceived as a failure?' *British Journal of Psychiatry 179,* 381–383.

Levinsky, N.G. (1996) 'The purpose of advance planning – autonomy for patients or limitation of care.' *New England Journal of Medicine 335,* 741–743.

Lewis, J. (1999) 'The concepts of community care and primary care in the UK: the 1960s to the 1990s.' *Health and Social Care in the Community 7,* 333–341.

Locke, J. (1689/1948) *An Essay Concerning Human Understanding.* Abridged and edited Wilburn, R. London: J.M. Dent and Sons.

Lothian, J. (2006) 'Birth plans: the good, the bad and the future.' *Journal of Obstetrics, Gynaecology and Neonatal Nursing 35,* 295–303.

Lundgren, I., Berg, M., Lindmark, G. (2003) 'Is the childbirth experience improved by a birth plan?' *Journal of Midwifery and Women's Health 48,* 322–328.

Lynsen, J. (2006) 'Maryland advance directives forms now available.' www.washington blade.com/2006/7–27/news/localnews/md.cfm

Manic Depression Fellowship (undated) *Planning Ahead for People with Manic Depression.* London: MDF.

Martyn, S. (1994) 'Substituted judgement, best interests, and the need for best respect.' *Cambridge Quarterly of Healthcare Ethics 3,* 195–208.

Mazur, D.J. (2006) 'How successful are we at protecting preferences? Consent, informed consent, advance directives and substituted judgement.' *Medical Decision Making 26,* 106–109.

McCrone, J. (1993) *The Myth of Irrationality. The Science of Mind from Plato to Star Trek.* London: Macmillan.

McHaffie, H.E. (2005) *Vacant Possession. A Story of Proxy Decision Making.* Oxford: Radcliffe Publishing.

Mill, J.S. (1859/1969) *On Liberty.* In Warnock, M. (ed.) *Utilitarianism, including Mills on Liberty and Essay on Bentham.* London: Fontana.

Mill, J.S. (1861/1969) *Utilitarianism.* In Warnock, M. (ed.) *Utilitarianism, including Mills on Liberty and Essay on Bentham.* London: Fontana.

Molloy, D.W., Guyatt, G.H., Russo, R., Goeree, R. *et al.* (2000) 'Systematic implementation of an advance directive program in a nursing home.' *Journal of the American Medical Association 283,* 1437–1444.

Monahan, J., Bonnie, R.J., Appelbaum, P.S., Hyde, P.S. *et al.* (2001) 'Mandated Community Treatment.' *Psychiatric Services 52,* 1192–1205.

Moorhouse, A., Weisstub, D.N. (1996) 'Advance directives for research: ethical problems and responses.' *International Journal of Law and Psychiatry 19,* 107–141.

Morton, A. (2004) *On Evil.* London: Routledge.

Mueser, K., Bond, G., Drake, R., Resnick, S. (1998) 'Models of community care for severe mental illness: a review of research on case management.' *Schizophrenia Bulletin 24,* 37–74.

Munby, J. (1998) 'Rhetoric and reality: the limitations of patient self-determination in contemporary English law.' *Journal of Contemporary Health Law and Policy 14*, 315–334.

Muthappan, P., Forster, H., Wendler, D. (2005) 'Research advance directives; protection or obstacle?' *American Journal of Psychiatry 162*, 2389–2391.

National Resource Centre on Psychiatric Advance Directives (2006) *Psychiatric Advance Directives. How To Be Your Own Advocate.* NRC is a collaboration between Duke University, North Carolina, and Bazelon Center, Washington DC. www.nrc-pad.org/

National Schizophrenia Fellowship (2001) *A Question of Choice.* London: National Schizophrenia Fellowship.

National Schizophrenia Fellowship (Scotland) (1997) 'Local hero.' *NSF(Scotland) Newsletter, Summer*, 9.

Nozick, R. (1981) *Philosophical Explanations.* Cambridge, Massachusetts: Harvard University Press.

Nozick, R. (1993) *The Nature of Rationality.* Princeton, New Jersey: Princeton University Press.

Nuffield Council on Bioethics (2006) *Public Health: Ethical Issues.* London: NCB.

Papageorgiou, A., King, M., Janmohamed, A., Davidson, O. (2002) 'Advance directives for patients compulsorily admitted to hospital with serious mental illness.' *British Journal of Psychiatry 181*, 513–519.

Papageorgiou, A., Janmohamed, A., King, M., Davidson, O. (2004) 'Advance directives for patients compulsorily admitted to hospital with serious mental illness: Directive content and feedback from patients and professionals.' *Journal of Mental Health 13*, 379–388.

Parfit, D. (1984) *Reasons and Persons.* Oxford: Clarendon Press.

Parry-Jones, L. (1972) *The Trade in Lunacy.* London: Routledge.

Pears, D. (1986) *Motivated Irrationality.* Oxford: Oxford University Press.

Perry, C., Quinn, L., Lindemann Nelson, J. (2002) 'Birth plans and professional autonomy.' *Hastings Centre Report 32*, 12–13.

Peters, C., Chiverton, P. (2003) 'Use of a values history in approaching medical advance directives with psychiatric patients.' *Journal of Psychosocial Nursing 41*, 28–36.

Pilgrim, D. (2005) 'Protest and co-option – the voice of mental health service users.' In Bell, A., Lindley, P. (eds) *Beyond the Water Towers. The Unfinished Revolution in Mental Health Services 1985–2005.* London: Sainsbury Centre for Mental Health.

Pilgrim, D., Waldron, L. (1998) 'User involvement in mental health services: how far can it go?' *Journal of Mental Health 7*, 95–104.

Porter, R. (1990) *Mind-Forg'd Manacles. A History of Madness in England from the Restoration to the Regency.* London: Penguin.

Potts, L. (2005) 'Patients get greater control over treatment.' Santa Cruz County, USA: National Alliance for the Mentally Ill. www.namiscc.org/Advocacy/2005/winter/usingadvance directives.htm

Priaulx, E. (2003) 'Enforcing advance directives. P&As assist individuals to retain self-determination in times of mental health crisis.' *Protection and Advocacy News 1.* www.napas.org/pub/PANews/0303advdir.htm

Promoting Excellence (undated) 'End-of-life care for persons with serious mental illness.' www.mywhatever.com/cifwriter/library/41/pe1251.html

Pruchno, R.A., Lemay, E.P.Jr, Feild, L., Levinsky, N.G. (2006) 'Predictors of patient treatment preferences and spouse substituted judgements: the case of dialysis continuation.' *Medical Decision Making 26*, 112–121.

Rachels, J. (1986) *The Elements of Moral Philosophy*. New York: McGraw Hill.

Rapaport, J. (2004) 'A matter of principle: the nearest relative under the Mental Health Act 1983 and proposals for legislative reform.' *Journal of Social Welfare and Family Law 26*, 377–396.

Rapaport, J. (2005) 'The informal caregiving experience: issues and dilemmas.' In Ramon, S., Williams, J.E. (eds) *Mental Health at the Crossroads: the Promise of the Professional Approach*. Aldershot: Ashgate.

Read, J., Baker, S. (1996) *Not Just Sticks and Stone: A Survey of the Discrimination Experienced by People with Mental Health Problems*. London: Mind.

Rethink (2000) *Policy Statements 25 and 26*. Kingston-on-Thames: Rethink. www.rethink.org/how_we_can_help/campaigning_for_change/rethink_policy_documents/index.html

Reznek, L. (1997) *Evil or Ill? Justifying the Insanity Defence*. London: Routledge.

Rhoden, N.K. (1982) 'Commentary on Winston, M.E. and Winston S.M. Can a subject consent to a "Ulysses contract"?' *Hastings Centre Report 12*, 26–28.

Richter, J., Eisemann, R.J. (1999) 'The compliance of doctors and nurses with do-not resuscitate orders in Germany and Sweden.' *Resuscitation 42*, 203–209.

Ritchie, J., Sklar, R., Steiner, W. (1998) 'Advance directives in psychiatry. Resolving issues of autonomy and competence.' *International Journal of Law and Psychiatry 21*, 245–260.

Rissmiller, D.J., Rissmiller, J.H. (2006) 'Evolution of the antipsychiatric movement into mental health consumerism.' *Psychiatric Services 57*, 863–866.

Roberts, G., Wolfson, P. (2004) 'The rediscovery of recovery: open to all.' *Advances in Psychiatric Treatment 10*, 37–49.

Rogers, A., Pilgrim, D. (1991) 'Pulling down churches: accounting for the mental health users' movement.' *Sociology of Mental Health and Illness 13*, 129–148.

Rogers A., Pilgrim, D. (1994) *Mental Health Policy in Britain*. Basingstoke: Macmillan.

Rogers, J.A., Centifanti, J.B. (1991) 'Beyond "self-paternalism": Response to Rosenson and Kasten.' *Schizophrenia Bulletin 17*, 9–14.

Romme, M., Escher, S. (2000) *Hearing Voices*. London: Mind.

Rosenson, M.K., Kasten, A.M. (1991) 'Another view of autonomy: Arranging to consent in advance.' *Schizophrenia Bulletin 17*, 1–7.

Rudnick, A. (2002) 'Depression and competence to refuse psychiatric treatment.' *Journal of Medical Ethics 28*, 151–158.

Ryle, G. (1963) '*The Concept of Mind*.' Harmondsworth: Penguin.

Sachs, S.G. (1994) 'Advance consent for dementia research.' *Alzheimer's Disease and Associated Disorders 8*, supplement 4, 19–27.

Sachs, G.A., Stocking, C.B., Stern, R., Cox., D.M. *et al.* (1994) 'Ethical aspects of dementia research: informed consent and proxy consent.' *Clinical Research 42*, 403–412.

Sainsbury Centre for Mental Health (2005) *Back on Track? CPA Care Planning for Service Users Who Are Repeatedly Detained Under the Mental Health Act*. London: Sainsbury Centre for Mental Health.

Sainsbury Centre for Mental Health (2006) *Choice in Mental Health Care*. Briefing 31. London: Sainsbury Centre for Mental Health.

Sales, G. (1993) 'The health care proxy for mental illness: can it work and should we want it?' *Bulletin of the Academy of Psychiatry and the Law 21*, 161–179.

Savulescu, J., Dickenson, D. (1998a) 'The time frame of preferences, dispositions, and the validity of advance directives for the mentally ill.' *Philosophy, Psychiatry and Psychology 5*, 225–246.

Savulescu, J., Dickenson, D. (1998b) 'Response to the Commentaries.' *Philosophy, Psychiatry and Psychology 5*, 263–266.

Sayce, L. (2000) *From Psychiatric Patient to Citizen: Overcoming Discrimination and Social Exclusion.* Basingstoke: Macmillan.

Schirm, V., Stachel, L. (1996) 'The values history as a nursing intervention to encourage use of advance directives among older adults.' *Applied Nursing Research 9*, 93–96.

Scott-Moncrieff, L. (2005) 'A sense of "déjà vu" – a preliminary (and immediate) response to the report of the Scrutiny Committee on the draft Mental Health Bill.' *Journal of Mental Health Law 12*, 77–82.

Scottish Executive (2001) *New Directions: Report on the Review of the Mental Health (Scotland) Act 1984 (Millan Report).* Edinburgh: Scottish Executive.

Scottish Executive (2003) *An Introduction to the Mental Health (Care and Treatment) (Scotland) Act 2003.* Edinburgh: Scottish Executive.

Scottish Executive (2004) *The New Mental Health Act. A Guide to Advance Statements.* Edinburgh: Scottish Executive.

Scottish Executive (2005) *Mental Health (Care and Treatment) (Scotland) Act 2003 Code of Practice.* Vols 1,2,3. Edinburgh: Scottish Executive.

Scottish Parliament (2002) *Health and Community Committee, Wednesday 30 October 2002.* Edinburgh: Stationery Office.

Scottish Parliament (2003) *Mental Health (Care and Treatment) (Scotland) Act 2003.* Edinburgh: Stationery Office.

Scull, A.T. (1982) *Museums of Madness. The Social Organisation of Insanity in Nineteenth Century England.* Harmondsworth: Penguin.

Seckler, A.B., Meirer, M.E., Mulvihill, M., Paris, B.E. (1991) 'Substituted judgement; how accurate are proxy predictions?' *Annals of Internal Medicine 115*, 743–745.

Shalowitz, D.I., Garrett-Meyer, E., Wendler, D. (2006) 'The accuracy of surrogate decision makers. A systematic review.' *Archives of Internal Medicine 166*, 493–497.

Sherman, P.S. (1998) 'Computer-assisted creation of psychiatric advance directives.' *Community Mental Health Journal 34*, 351–362.

Shore, D. (2006) 'Ethical issues in schizophrenia research: A commentary on some concerns.' *Schizophrenia Bulletin 32*, 26–29.

Shorter, E. (1997) *A History of Psychiatry from the Era of the Asylum to the Age of Prozac.* New York: Wiley.

Showalter, E. (1987) *The Female Malady. Women, Madness and English Culture 1830–1980.* London: Virago.

Shumway, M., Saunders, T., Shern, D., Pines, E. (2003) 'Preferences for schizophrenia treatment outcomes among public policy makers, consumers, families and providers.' *Psychiatric Services 54*, 1124–1128.

Simpson, A., Miller, C., Powers, I. (2003a) 'Case management. Models and the Care Programme Approach: How to make the CPA creditable and effective.' *Journal of Psychiatric and Mental Health Nursing 10*, 472–483.

Simpson, A., Miller, C., Powers, I. (2003b) 'The history of the Care Programme Approach in England: Where did it go wrong?' *Journal of Mental Health 12*, 489–504.

Smiley, M. (1992) *Moral Responsibility and the Boundaries of Community*. Chicago: University of Chicago Press.

Smith, D.G., Nunn, S. (1995) 'Commentary on substituted judgement: in search of a foolproof method; A response to Baergin.' *Journal of Clinical Ethics 6*, 184–186.

Srebnik, D., Appelbaum, P.S., Russo, J. (2004) 'Assessing competence to complete psychiatric advance directives with the competence assessment tool for psychiatric advance directives.' *Comprehensive Psychiatry 45*, 239–245.

Srebnik, D., Brodoff, L. (2003) 'Implementing psychiatric advance directives: service provider issues and answers.' *Journal of Behavioural Health Services and Research 30*, 253–268.

Srebnik, D.S., Kim, S.Y. (2006) 'Competency for creation, use and revocation of psychiatric advance directives.' *Journal of the American Academy of Psychiatry and Law 34*, 501–510.

Srebnik, D.S., Russo, J., Sage, J., Peto, T. *et al.* (2003) 'Interest in psychiatric advance directives among high users of crisis services and hospitalisation.' *Psychiatric Services 54*, 981–986.

Srebnik, D.S., Rutherford, L.T., Peto, T., Russo, J. *et al.* (2005) 'The content and clinical utility of psychiatric advance directives.' *Psychiatric Services 56*, 592–598.

Stanhope, J. (2006) 'Medical treatment direction will protect rights of patients.' Media release. www.chiefminister.act.gov.au/media.asp?media=1915&section=52&title=medi

Stavis, P.F. (1993) 'The Health Care Proxy Law: Is it a "catch 22" for many persons with mental illness?' *Quality of Care Newsletter 57*. www.cqc.state.ny.us/counsels_corner/cc57.htm

Stavis, P.E. (1999) 'The Nexum: a modest proposal for self-guardianship by contract; a system of advance directives and surrogate committees-at-large for the intermittently mentally ill.' *Journal of Contemporary Health Law Policy 16*, 1–95.

Steadman, H.J., Gounis, K., Dennis, D., Hopper, K. *et al.* (2001) 'Assessing the New York involuntary outpatient community Pilot Programme.' *Psychiatric Services 52*, 1533–1534.

Stein, I., Test, M. (1980) 'Alternatives to mental hospital treatment, 1. Conceptual model, treatment programme and clinical evaluation.' *Archives of General Psychiatry 37*, 392–397.

Stocking, C.B., Hougham, G.W., Danner, D.D., Patterson, M.B. (2006) 'Speaking of research advance directives: planning for future research participation.' *Neurology 9*, 1361–1366.

Sturdee, P.G. (1995) 'Irrationality and the dynamic unconscious: the case for wishful thinking.' *Philosophy, Psychiatry and Psychology 2*, 163–174.

Suhl, J., Simmons, P., Reedy, T., Garrick, T. (1994) 'Myth of substituted judgement. Surrogate decision making regarding life support is unreliable.' *Archives of Internal Medicine 154*, 90–96.

Sullivan, D., Szmuckler, G. (2001) 'Psychiatric advance directives.' *Schizophrenia Monitor 11*, 1–4.

Sutherby, K., Henderson, C., Flood, C. (2004) 'Training pack for the development of a joint crisis plan.' www.bmj.com/cgi/content/full/bmj.38155.585046.63/DC1

Sutherby, K., Szmuckler, G.H., Halpern, A., Alexander, M. (1999) 'A study of "crisis cards" in a community psychiatric service.' *Acta Psychiatrica Scandinavia 100*, 56–61.

Sutherland, S. (1992) *Irrationality. Why We Don't Think Straight!* New Brunswick: Rutgers University Press.

Swanson, J.W., Tepper, M.C., Backlar, P., Swartz, M.S. (2000) 'Psychiatric advance directives: An alternative to coercive treatment?' *Psychiatry 63*, 160–172.

Swanson, J.W., Van McCrary, S., Swartz, M.S., Elbogen, E.B. *et al.* (2006a) 'Superseding psychiatric advance directives: Ethical and legal considerations.' *Journal of the American Academy of Psychiatry and Law 84*, 385–394.

Swanson, J.W., Swartz, M.S., Elbogen, E.B., Van Dorn, R.A. *et al.* (2006c) 'Facilitated psychiatric advance directives: A randomised trial of an intervention to foster advance treatment planning among persons with severe mental illness.' *American Journal of Psychiatry 163*, 1943–1951.

Swanson, J.W., Swartz, M.S., Ferron, J., Elbogen, E. *et al.* (2006b) 'Psychiatric advance directives among public mental health consumers in five U.S. cities: prevalence, demand and correlates.' *Journal of the American Academy of Psychiatry and Law 34*, 43–57.

Swanson, J.W., Swartz, M.S., Hannon, M.J., Elbogen, E.B. *et al.* (2003) 'Psychiatric advance directives: a survey of persons with schizophrenia, family members, and treatment providers.' *International Journal of Forensic Mental Health 2*, 73–86.

Swanson, J.W., Van McCrary, S., Swartz, M.S., Van Dorn, R.A. *et al.* (2007) 'Overriding psychiatric advance directives: Factors associated with psychiatric decisions to pre-empt patients' advance refusal of hospitalisation and medication.' *Law and Human Behaviour* 31, 277–290.

Swartz, M.S., Swanson, J.W. (2004) 'Involuntary outpatient commitment, community treatment orders and associated outpatient treatment: What's in the data.' *Canadian Journal of Psychiatry 49*, 585–591.

Swartz, M.S., Swanson, J.W., Ferron, J., Elbogen, E.B. *et al.* (2005) 'Psychiatrists' views and attitudes about psychiatric advance directives.' *International Journal of Forensic Mental Health 4*, 107–117.

Swartz, M.S., Swanson, J.W., Van Dorn, R.A., Elbogen, E.B. *et al.* (2006) 'Patient preferences for psychiatric advance directives.' *International Journal of Forensic Mental Health 5*, 67–81.

Szasz, T.S. (1961) *The Myth of Mental Illness: Foundations of a Theory of Personal Conduct.* New York: Hoeber-Harper.

Szasz, T.S. (1963) *Law, Liberty and Psychiatry: An Inquiry into the School Uses of Mental Health Practices.* New York: Macmillan.

Szasz, T.S. (1979) *The Myth of Psychotherapy: Mental Healing as Rhetoric, Religion and Repression.* New York: Doubleday.

Szasz, T.S. (1982) 'The psychiatric will. A new mechanism for protecting persons against "psychosis" and psychiatry.' *American Psychologist 37*, 762–770.

Szmukler, G., Dawson, J. (2006) 'Commentary: Towards resolving some dilemmas concerning psychiatric advance directives.' *Journal of the American Academy of Psychiatry and the Law 34*, 398–401.

Tait, L., Lester, H. (2005) 'Encouraging user involvement in mental health services.' *Advances in Psychiatric Treatment 11*, 168–175.

Tan, J., Hope, A., Stewart, A. (2003) 'Competence to refuse treatment in anorexia nervosa.' *International Journal of Law and Psychiatry 26*, 697–707.

Taylor, D., Tan, S-L. (2000) 'Advance directives knowledge and research appears lacking in Australia.' *Emergency Medicine 12*, 255–256.

Taylor, J., Laurie, S., Geddes, J. (1996) 'Factors associated with admission to hospital following emergency psychiatric assessment.' *Health Bulletin 54*, 467–473.

Teno, J.M. (2000) 'Advance directives for nursing home residents: achieving compassionate, competent, cost effective care.' *Journal of the American Medical Association 283*, 1481–1482.

Thomas, P. (1997) *The Dialectics of Schizophrenia.* London: Free Association Books.

Thomas, P. (2003) 'How should advance statements be implemented?' *British Journal of Psychiatry 182*, 548–549.

Thomas, P.T., Cahill, A.B. (2004) 'Compulsion and psychiatry – the role of advance statements.' *British Medical Journal 329*, 122–123.

Tomlinson, T., Howe, K., Notman, M., Rossmiller, D. (1990) 'An empirical study of proxy consent for elderly persons.' *The Gerentologist 30*, 54–64.

Tsevat, J., Cook, E.F., Green. M.L., Matcher, D.B. *et al.* (1995) 'Health values of the seriously ill.' *Annals of Internal Medicine 122*, 514–520.

Turner, T.H. (2004) 'Compulsory treatment can be liberating.' *British Medical Journal 329*, Rapid response. www.bmj.com/cgi/eletters/329/7458/122

Unsworth, C. (1987) *Politics of Mental Health Legislation.* Oxford: Clarendon Press.

Upadya, A., Muralidharan, V., Thorevska, N., Amoeteng-Adjepong, Y. (2002) 'Physician and family member understanding of living wills.' *American Journal of Respiratory and Critical Care Medicine 166*, 1430–1435.

Valleto, N.M., Kamahele, R., Menon, A.S., Ruskin, P. (2002) 'Completion of advance directives for general health care among inpatients with schizophrenia.' *Journal of Nervous and Mental Disease 190*, 264–265.

Van Dorn, R., Swartz, M.S., Elbogen, C.B., Swanson, J.W. *et al. (2006) 'Clinicians' attitudes regarding barriers to the implementation of psychiatric advance directives.' Administration and Policy in Mental Health and Mental Health Services 33*, 449–460.

Van Staden, C.W., Krüger, C. (2003) 'Incapacity to give informed consent owing to mental disorder.' *Journal of Medical Ethics 29*, 41–43.

Van Willigenburg, T., Delaere, P. (2005) 'Protecting autonomy as authenticity using Ulysses contracts.' *Journal of Medical Philosophy 30*, 395–409.

Vuckovich, P.K. (2003) 'Psychiatric advance directives.' *Journal of the American Psychiatric Nurses Association 9*, 55–59.

Wallace, R.J. (1994) *Responsibility and the Moral Sentiments.* Cambridge, Massachusetts: Harvard University Press.

Wallcraft, J., Read, J., Sweeney, A. (2003) *On Our Own Terms: Users and Survivors of Mental Health Services Working Together for Support and Change.* London: Sainsbury Centre for Mental Health.

Washington State Department of Social and Health Services (2004) *Mental Health Advance Directives. Information for Consumers.*

Washington State Hospital Association (undated) *What Patients Need to Know About Mental Health Advance Directives.*

Watson, G. (1987) 'Responsibility and the limits of evil. Variations on a Strawsonian theme.' In Schoeman, F. (ed.) *Responsibility, Character and the Emotions.* Cambridge: Cambridge University Press.

Wauchope, B.R. (2006) *Implementing Advance Agreements into Mental Health Treatment and Care Planning: A Pilot Evaluation of the Process and Outcomes.* Unpublished PhD thesis for Doctor of Psychology (Clinical), Australian National University.

Whitford, H., Hillan, E. (1998) 'Women's perceptions of the birth plan.' *Midwifery 14*, 248–253.

Wiggins, D. (1967) *Identity and Spatio-temporal Continuity.* Oxford: Blackwell.

Wiggins, D. (1980) *Sameness and Substance.* Oxford: Oxford University Press.

Williams, B. (1973) *Problem of Self.* Cambridge: Cambridge University Press.

Winick, B.J. (1996) 'Advance directive instruments for those with mental illness.' *University of Miami Law Review 51*, 57–95.

Winick, B.J. (1997) *The Right to Refuse Mental Health Treatment.* Washington: American Psychiatric Association.

Winston, M., Winston, S., Appelbaum, P., Rhoden, N. (1982) 'Can a subject consent to a Ulysses contract? Commentary.' *Hastings Centre Report 12*, 27–28.

Wolf, S. (1987) 'Sanity and the metaphysics of responsibility.' In Schoeman, F. (ed.) *Responsibility, Character and the Emotions.* Cambridge: Cambridge University Press.

Wolfe, J., Gournay, K., Norman, S., Ramnoruth, D. (1997) 'Care Programme Approach: Evaluation of its implications in an inner London service.' *Clinical Effectiveness in Nursing 1*, 85–91.

Wong, J.G., Clare, I.C.H., Gunn, M.J., Holland, A.J. (1999) 'Capacity to make health care decisions; its importance in clinical practice.' *Psychological Medicine 29*, 437–446.

World Health Organisation (2005) *WHO Resource Book on Mental Health, Human Rights and Legislation.* Geneva: WHO.

World Health Organisation Department of Reproductive Health and Research (1999) *Care in Normal Birth: A Practical Guide.* Geneva: WHO.

Useful websites

Scotland
Mental Health (Care and Treatment) (Scotland) Act 2003
www.opsi.gov.uk/legislation/scotland/acts2003/20030013.htm
Direct access to the Mental Health (Care and Treatment) (Scotland) Act 2003.

www.scotland.gov.uk/Topics/Health/health/mental-health/mhlaw/home
This website provides advice and guidance on the Act, as well as links to the legislation and its associated regulations.

www.scotland.gov.uk/Publications/2004/10/20017/44081
Direct link to guide to advance statements.

Mental Welfare Commission for Scotland
www.mwcscot.org.uk/home/home.asp
The Mental Welfare Commission for Scotland is an independent organisation working to safeguard the rights and welfare of everyone with a mental illness, learning disability or other mental disorder. For information and advice.

England and Wales
Mental Health Act Commission
www.mhac.org.uk/
The Mental Health Act Commission reviews the Mental Health Act 1983 and safeguards the rights of people subject to the Act.

Mind
www.mind.org.uk/index.htm
Direct link to Mind's briefing on advance directives.

USA

SAMHSA

http://mentalhealth.samhsa.gov/cmhs/PAIMI

This is a link to Protection and Advocacy for Individuals with Mental illness Program (PAIMI) which gives information on state laws.

Duke University

http://pad.duhs.duke.edu/background.html

Provides information on the Duke University Programme on Advance Directives.

National Resource Centre on Psychiatric Advance Directives

www.nrc-pad.org/

This is the National Resource Centre on Psychiatric Advance Directives – for details on all state laws in relation to advance directives.

Bazelon Centre

http://bazelon.org/

This describes the Bazelon Centre for Mental Health Law – information and advocacy.

National Alliance on Mental Illness

http://nami.org/

This is the National Alliance on Mental Illness commentary on advance directives.

Glossary

ADA	Americans with Disabilities Act
CPA	Care Programme Approach
CPN	Community psychiatric nurse
CTO	Community treatment order
DNR	Do not resuscitate
DPA/DPOA	Durable power of attorney
ECT	Electro-convulsive therapy
EPA	Enduring power of attorney
NHS	National Health Service
PAD	Psychiatric advance directive
PRA	Principle of responsive adjustment
PVS	Persistent vegetative state
RMO	Responsible medical officer
SW	Social work(er)
WHO	World Health Organisation

Subject Index

Author Index